The Voyage of Love & Sex

Best wishes

Diane Sommer.

25 Sept 2004

Acknowledgements

I could not have taken on this task without learning to face the challenges of my own voyage from everyone who has touched my life.

I would like to acknowledge Rosemary Allan who encouraged me to develop my writing style and gave much needed editorial advice. I also had magnificent professional support from Olga Eyles.

The Voyage of Love & Sex

Dr Diane Summer

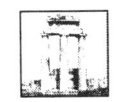

THE ORACLE PRESS

Published by The Oracle Press
P.O. Box 121 Montville Qld 4560 Australia

All rights reserved. No part of this book,
either in part or in whole, may be reproduced,
transmitted or utilised in any form, by any means,
electronic, photographic or mechanical, including photocopying,
recording or by any information storage system, without permission
in writing from the publisher, except for brief quotations
embodied in literary articles and reviews.

©Diane Summer, 1999

National Library of Australia
ISBN: 1 876494 07 7

Front cover: Pastel by Lynn Cran

Printed by Watson Ferguson & Co., Moorooka, Queensland 4105

Preface

I have been privileged to know clients, colleagues, friends and family who have opened their hearts to discuss intimate aspects of them Selves. They honestly related their own voyages through the problems and passions of love. From them I learned that love of Self and of Others is an essential part of happiness. Some discovered the joy of human sexuality in the presence of a beloved and were enriched. They have been the greatest influence on my work as a doctor and therapist in sexual relationships. They developed my knowledge which I want to share.

> *Sex to me means the whole of the relationship*
> *between man and woman...*
> *And the relation of man to woman is as wide as life...*
> *The relationship is a lifelong change*
> *and a lifelong travelling...*
> *At periods the sex-desire itself departs completely.*
> *Yet the flow of the relationship goes*
> *on all the same, undying*
> *And that is the flow of living sex.*
>
> D. H. Lawrence

Contents

Introduction — 10

Part One
Preparing for the Voyage

1. Is it lust or love? — 19
  Drive
  Desire
  Why do you have sex?

2. Boy meets girl — 29
  Biological difference
  Roles assigned by gender
  Problem solving
  Styles of intimacy
  Understanding and appreciating difference

3. Who makes the rules? — 41
  Culture and religion in the past
  Your choice in the present

4. Lessons and teachers — 51
  Family
  Positive learning
  Negative learning
  School
  Self exploration
  Sexual abuse
  Reaching your potential

5. *Only flesh and blood?*   63
    Hormones
    Blood circulation
    Nerve connections
    State of mind
    Body image

6. *What is this thing called love?*   81
    Unconditional love
    Dependent love
    Provisional love
    Mature love
    Dysfunctional love
    Making love
    Divine love
    What do you mean by love?

Part Two
Embarking on the Love Boat

7. *The honeymoon suite*   97
    Essentials of 'in love'
    Saying what you really feel with honesty and tact
    Positive signals for continuing from 'in love'

8. *Fog warning*   115
    Sharing love or needing a relationship?
    Differences between needing and sharing

Part Three
Troubled Waters

9. Out of the mist — 129
- Awareness of differences
- Compatibility
- Separating
- Staying longer
- Win/lose
- Open conflict

10. All at sea — 147
- Hidden conflict
- Unhealthy compromise
- Sex in troubled waters
- Beyond troubled waters

11. The voyage becomes a challenge — 161
- Why does a relationship 'go wrong'
- Incompatibility
- The pressures of life
- Difference
- Fixed roles
- Behaviour patterns
- Self esteem
- Disappointment in love and sex
- The challenge of relationship

Part Four
Charting New Waters

12. Changing course — 185
- Considering change
- Updating childhood learning
- Respectful discussion
- When one says 'No'

13. Becalmed — 205
Respect for difference
Fundamental difference
What is Self with a capital 'S'?
Being your Self versus selfish
Losing your Self
Self sacrifice or Self care
Releasing your Self
Who am I?

14. The wind in your sails — 221
Independence
Interdependence
Your Self in sex
The Red Shoes

Part Five
The Shores of the Heart

15. Ebb and flow — 235
Intimate desires
Reaching your potential
Sensuality

16. Skinny-dipping — 255
Erotica or pornography
Fantasy

17. Dawn on the horizon — 265
Mature love and sex
Body/spirit mind-blowing orgasm
Divine sex
Unconditional touch

References — 274

Introduction

Did you embark on the voyage of love and sex buoyant with hope and joy? But over time have your feelings ebbed and flowed. Do you wonder why happiness seems more distant than when you set sail? Why are there problems with love? Why is sex different now? What course should you chart to find the fulfilment you seek?

Many popular books, magazines and movies would have you believe that a sure-fire formula for 'happiness ever after' is simply love plus the natural urge for sex. But something inside you knows that the love boat is powered by more than lust alone. Your own experience of a long-term relationship rarely matches the myth that sexual sharing is an easy, automatic and unchanging condition. Instead you find relationships go through different stages which are naturally reflected in your responses and feelings.

In reality many people will experience variations in love and sex, wanting more, wanting less, or not at all, a different partner, problems with erection, not getting an orgasm or having one too quickly or too slowly.

If you turn to medical books for an explanation you find the words 'Sexual Dysfunction' used to describe these fluctuations, giving the impression that the body is not working well. But we are more than bodies alone.

The World Health Organisation defines health as 'a state of dynamic harmony between the body, mind and spirit of a person and the social and cultural influences which make up his or her environment.' I realised, as I listened to the experiences of my clients, how relevant this approach is to understanding sexuality. I believe that many people are functioning normally as thinking, feeling human beings when they have a problem with sex. They are expressing through their bodies the problems of their relationship, their upbringing, their beliefs, their health – their whole self.

This is not to suggest that problems should be ignored. On the contrary, feeling uncomfortable with sex can generate much concern. But discomfort can have the benefit of making you take a fresh look at these areas of your life. An opportunity is presented to develop a loving intimacy with your self and your beloved.

The Voyage of Love & Sex helps you navigate the calm and storms that real relationships encounter. It will help you resolve difficulties, be they big or small, to find a sustainable happiness. Of course this is not a luxury cruise and some of the problems will be challenging.

People came to see me for help with such problems. In my professional life I started out like any conventional doctor when presented with sexual difficulties, by offering prescriptions to cure hormone imbalance, boost desire, etc. But I found such treatments were insufficient for many problems. I realised that to truly help my clients I needed to know more than I had learned in medical school. Subsequently I trained in relationship counselling and sex therapy. I added to this the wealth of experience of my clients, colleagues, psychologists and philosophers who helped expand my understanding.

Amongst the first books I read were the works of the pioneers in the field of sex therapy. In the 1960s Masters and Johnson reported on their new work using 'Sensate Focus'. They recommended that couples relearn sensitive touching of the body (particularly the genitals). The focus was on the 'doing' of sex. Their two-week residential courses had 'successes'. But such successes proved to be temporary. When the couples returned to their usual home and work environment difficulties with sex recurred. Clearly a course in sensual touching, however pleasant that can be, is insufficient.

As I worked, studied and lived, I found myself increasingly recognising the importance of thoughts, emotions and heart-felt love, as well as the body, in sexuality. We are coming to appreciate that their separation has resulted in an incomplete understanding of human love and sex.

Scientific research helped to explain the physical part of sex. Blood vessels, nerve endings, erections, vaginal lubrication and orgasms have all been described in the textbooks. But that is not all there is to sex.

Religious sources contributed on the spiritual side. Unfortunately in Western culture, sex was seen as sinful for centuries. We were led to feel guilty about the human joy of sexual pleasure, which did more harm than good.

Early psychologists made assumptions about the mind in sex. They confused us even more. Were we normal to enjoy (or not enjoy) sex, or were we suffering neuroses?

We need to integrate these intrinsic parts of love and sex to feel fulfilled. Yet we overlooked this essential truth for a long time.

During their first consultation many of my clients said their only discontent was in the physical performance of sex. As they talked, many (both men and women) began to reveal the emptiness and disappointment they felt in their sexual lives. Many had known joy with sex at some time in their life, often at the beginning of a

INTRODUCTION

relationship, but now found dissatisfaction associated with sex.

Have you ever dismissed a problem by blaming it on a physical cause alone? 'Sex was fine until we had the baby, menopause, the Pill, blood pressure', the list goes on. These are all relevant but usually there is much more involved. It is tempting to look for 'quick fix' solutions to sexual problems but they rarely help. You may have tried some – sexy lingerie, new positions, massaging your partner, etc. They can be fun when you are hot for each other, but who needs advice then!

When you are really concerned about sex, a sex manual, which offers 'quick fixes' can be such a disappointment. If you have been left wondering what is wrong with you, take heart. Maybe the suggestions were wrong – for you.

This book is for men and women who want clear understandable ideas to guide them through the complexity of real, sexual relationships. It will encourage you to trust your instinct that sexuality is not only physical but also embraces your thinking, feeling and your desire for intimacy. These uniquely human aspects of love and sex are as vital a part of this book as they are of you.

Part One, 'Preparing for the Voyage', briefly looks at the history of our present views on sexuality. It lets you explore what has influenced your own beliefs, about love and sex. Family, religion, culture, gender and personal experiences all contribute to your beliefs. Health and lifestyle also have an impact on how you express your self sexually. Your sexual relationships develop in the context of this broad background.

For many sex is part of the experience of love with another. Yet the word 'love' has many interpretations. The various concepts of love are defined to help you to recognise what you mean by the word 'love'. How do you associate love with sex? Why do you have sex? You will understand your own motivations when you complete the questionnaire at the end of this section.

You may find this background understanding not what you need right now. If you are anxious to get straight to the heart of your relationship you may prefer to skip to Part Two. (Part One can also be enjoyable after reaching the end of the book).

Part Two looks at love and sex in the first stage of a relationship – when you are 'embarking on the love boat'. Through the personal stories of two couples you can analyse what happens and why. They express the joys and problems of being 'in love'. Talking about what you want when 'in love' is a great idea. But not many go beyond 'everything is lovely' for fear of hurting the feelings of the other. You will recognise how and why you should talk honestly (including about sex).

A checklist called 'Positive signals for continuing from 'in love', helps you take stock of your relationship and assess compatibility.

Part Two also helps you to distinguish the difference between loving someone and needing them.

Part Three looks at the next phase of love and sex in 'Troubled Waters'. There are examples of couples who each navigate this time in different ways. You can share their problems and understand their reasons.

At some time you will encounter this stage in your relationship as the differences between your self and partner begin to be clearly seen. A confusion of feelings arises as you enter a time of disillusionment when difficulties and conflicts result.

This section looks at why a relationship 'goes wrong'. It comes as no surprise during stormy weather that the bedroom is no longer a haven.

Part Four entitled 'Charting New Waters', explores how the couples try to achieve respectful discussion of their inevitable differences. They find it is not easy to shift from the struggle of win/lose and blame – to respecting as equal the opinions of both. They discover though, this shift is essential for the health and survival of a relationship. The differences between your self and your partner challenge you to change.

The individuals presented as cases show how they cope with revealing their true thoughts and feelings. They learn to steer their way through their problems. Some find renewed pleasure with each other. With enjoyable effort their relationship and sexual desire blossoms once more.

For others, serious fundamental areas of incompatibility emerge which are recognised as unacceptable. They choose a different solution, which is still respectful of each other. Their experiences will help you decide what is right for you.

Part Four includes an essential section on self esteem. In the early part of your relationship your esteem may have been boosted by approval from your partner. These good feelings are dependent on your partner. This is not self-esteem but is esteem dependent on another. Some of our couples discover this early source of confidence can be lost once they hit troubled waters.

You too may have lost your sense of self in blending with your partner for the sake of the relationship. This is the time in a relationship that you can re-establish or develop for the first time self esteem and self respect.

'She/he is my other half' (wife/husband) is a common expression. 'In love' you may have thought you found your 'other half'. But being half a person is never enough. You can move beyond being two halves, to become two whole people who enjoy sharing your lives. You may find the exercise entitled, 'Who am I?', of particular help in this process.

In Part Five couples reach the 'The Shores of the Heart'. No longer all at sea, they feel the pleasure of being lapped by the waves of love and sex as they touch on solid ground. They appreciate the ebb and flow of life itself.

From understanding the changes in relationship over the years comes a deep sense of knowing your self and the other. Through the storms of troubled waters you grow as separate individuals and can be together from choice. You too can experience the joy of living up to your dreams not down to your fears. In the freedom of full expression of who you are, love continues to mature.

With hearts open to the delight of body, mind and spirit you find fulfilment in abundant intimacy on *The Voyage of Love & Sex*.

Life is an ocean, love is a boat,
In troubled waters it keeps us afloat.
Our true destination is not marked on any chart.
We're navigating for the shores of the heart.

'The Voyage'
Johnny Duhan

Part One

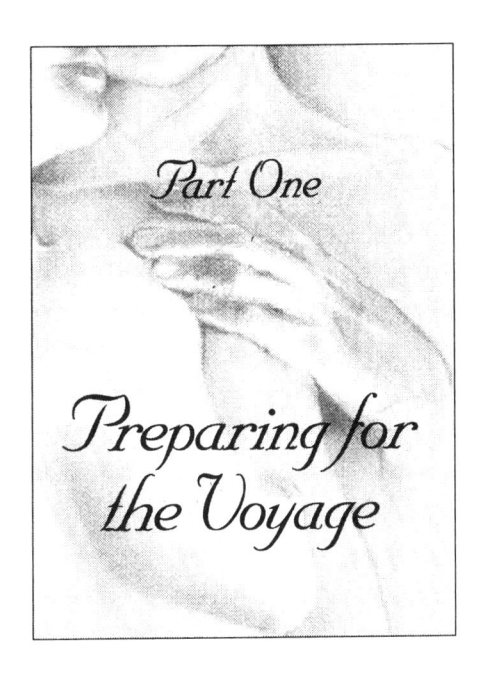

Preparing for the Voyage

Anticipation waits for love.
Will it be everything you dreamed?

'If We Fall In Love'
James Harris III
Terry Lewis

*Then you took the words right out of my mouth
It must have been while you were kissing me.
. . . and I swear it is true
I was just about to say 'I love you'.*

'You Took the Words Right Out of My Mouth'
Jim Steinman

Chapter One

Is it lust or love?

When you are looking for a mate to share your voyage it helps to find someone who speaks the same language. Unfortunately, the native tongue of sex is often assumed to be the same as the language of love. You will find the passage is easier if you understand each other's words.

Sexual drive, desire, arousal, lust, libido and love are all used in the context of sex. Are they the same? Does it matter what word you use? I think sexual drive and sexual desire are different. They have become confused and combined in the word 'libido'. I prefer not to use the word libido in this way as it has the richer and fuller meaning of 'impelling life force'. If you begin with separate definitions of drive and desire you can be clear about motives that underly sex. Love is an even bigger issue to which the whole of chapter six is devoted.

Sex drive is a basic urge. It is the same as lust. Hormones, particularly testosterone, act on the lower level of the brain to produce sex drive. Age changes, health problems and medications can also affect this level. This is the part of the brain which you have in common with animals so you can understand some of your behaviour from research in animals. But we are more than 'naked apes'[1] and are not only motivated by drive but also by desire.

Sexual desire is the human motivation for sex that involves thoughts and feelings. We have evolved beyond animals and possess an additional upper level of brain. This part of the brain is used to integrate thinking, emotions and memories which all contribute to the sex/love experience. Awareness of sexual desire is experienced using this upper level of brain.

Both drive and desire are potent motivators of sexual interest and neither should be disregarded. Both men and women have drive and desire. It may be that for men, as a result of their higher testosterone, drive may be more demanding of attention than it is in women.

There is nothing wrong with sex motivated by sex drive. We can all enjoy being animals sometimes. But satisfaction of drive alone expresses only one dimension of sexuality. It has its limits when sex is part of a long-term relationship.

In the turmoil of love and sex do you recognise if you and your partner have the same motivation? Is it drive or desire? Does lust become shrouded in words of love that can lead to all kinds of confusion and disappointment?

Justin (18) and Leanne (16) had been dating for a short while. Leanne recalled their last date. After a party they drove to a secluded spot and 'parked' for a while.

"He said I was gorgeous. We had some heavy kissing. When Justin touched me it was wonderful. He really turned me on. We got all heated up. He got a 'hard on'. I was kind of moist and all the windows were steamed up.

"Justin said, 'Do you want to have sex?' So I asked him, 'Do you love me?'

"'Oh Yes,' he said. But I wanted to hear him say it. When he said, 'I love you,' I just melted."

Was Justin in the throes of sex drive or desirous of sex with Leanne as he said, "I love you"? Leanne thought he was 'in love' with her, but when he did not telephone she was hurt and confused. They had not been talking the same language, and though they had used the same words each had a different meaning in mind. Leanne was motivated by desire for Justin as a result she felt sexy. Justin was motivated by his drive for sex with Leanne. Neither motivation is right or wrong. Problems arise from what is left unsaid about why you want sex.

It is not always easy to distinguish between drive and desire. The distinction becomes clearer by comparing sex to another basic of life – hunger. In both animals and man hunger is a very demanding drive. The drive to eat is essential for life.

The drive of hunger leads to a simple automatic response in animals. A dog for example will accept the same bowl of meat every night of the week. His basic hunger drive is easily satisfied. Try the same meal every night on your beloved and you will not be met with a wagging tail. He/she is more likely to be bored and refuse to eat the meal even if hungry.

You are more often motivated by the desire to eat rather than the drive of hunger. Human desire involves complex thinking. You consider your likes and dislikes. You may wonder about untried tastes and think of ways to create new flavours. You then add to this an extra ingredient – your mood. Whether you are happy, sad or excited determines whether you reach for a chocolate bar, eat an apple or eat nothing at all.

Humans are different in this way from many animals. In addition each human is different from others. Anxiety may cause you to make repeated raids on the fridge whilst someone else may lose their appetite. You want to grab fast food while your partner wants to savour a gourmet meal.

If you transfer this line of thought to sex you can appreciate that desire is a vital and complex influence on how you behave sexually. I think it is the overwhelming one in long-term relationships. The higher level of brain is affected by lifestyle, mood, personal relationships and childhood learning. The rich range of emotions that you feel is essential in understanding the full breadth of your sexual interest and responses.

The human context

You can learn the mechanics of sexuality from animal studies but it is only in the context of body, mind and spirit you appreciate the full human experience of sex.

If sexual intercourse was only about reproduction it might be as simple for you as it is for animals. But studies reveal that even human genitals are different from all other creatures. In animals, the vaginal opening is designed only for rear entry. During sexual intercourse the female can not see her partner. She may even appear disinterested in the whole process and carry on eating a banana. The male animal experiences ejaculation and then goes off to play or sleep. If you just thought 'we're not that different' - you can be.

You are a member of the only species on the planet in which the vagina faces forwards. As a result you have the opportunity to look at your partner during sex. You know with whom you are having sex. You see their face, their expression, read the emotion in their eyes and sense their mood. Human, face to face, sex has this additional dimension of intimate communication.

The second significant difference between humans and animals is that the female animal is not thought to experience orgasm, nor pleasure, during intercourse. The drive for sex in a female animal is the hormonal change, which makes her 'in season'. She is only able to conceive at this particular time and it is the only time she is sexually receptive. In the elephant this occurs only every four years. Clearly we are different. You (man or woman) are unique in that interest in sex is a possibility, though not necessarily your choice, every day of the year.

It is theorised that these two major differences of humans from animals confer an advantage in bonding a man and woman. We have moved beyond sex for reproduction, into the realm of relationships. When dreaming of a long-term connection your choice of partner is based not only on physical attraction, your feelings are also involved. This emotional link undoubtedly contributes to being able to contemplate the long haul of human child rearing and beyond.

The period of 'beyond' has extended considerably in recent years as you live longer than your ancestors. Not only do you want this extension of life to be healthier but also more fulfilling. As a major contributor to happiness you may view relationships in a new light. Staying together is no longer 'just for the children'. You may be seeking greater satisfaction and meaning in your life and find your self reviewing your attitude towards work, family, marriage or childrearing. To meet these challenges you need to overcome previous restrictions to find ways to reach your potential.

Part of the health and happiness you seek can be found in the intimacy of sexual pleasure. If you rely only on sex drive and its physical expression, this pleasure ends at orgasm. Disconnection of the body and mind can lead to the mere performance of sexual intercourse. It has satisfaction but also limits. On the other hand when intimate feelings direct the body you can find fulfilment of more than your sexual desire. The desire does not end with orgasm. The joy you feel fuels your desire for sexual sharing with your beloved in the future.

If you feel this explanation has made human sex sound complex. It is and you are. But through appreciating this complexity, you can arrive at simple personal truths. There is a simple grace in the sharing of sex and love by two mutually respecting human beings.

To reach this state requires your willingness to gain insight into your motives, hopes and dreams that you associate with love and sex. This can free you to have the confidence to fully open your self physically and emotionally to another.

Why do you have sex?

This may seem a ridiculously simple question, one you may not have asked your self before assuming there was only one answer. But as you glance through this list you may realise you have many reasons that change from day to day. They may derive from desire, drive, love or need.

Answer Yes or No to each statement from your own experience. It is not necessary to keep a score.

Why do you have sex?

- I find my partner attractive.
- I find my partner sexy.
- I feel 'horny' (turned on, aroused).
- I enjoy my body being caressed.
- To have an orgasm.
- I want a baby.
- I have been drinking alcohol.
- I have been smoking marijuana.
- To stop my partner having an affair.
- To stop my partner from leaving me.
- To be reassured that I am attractive.
- To prove my partner is mine.
- To forget my problems.
- To relieve my stress.
- To patch over an argument.
- He/she gets angry if I don't.

- He/she feels rejected if I don't.
- It stops me feeling bad about myself.
- Everyone else seems to enjoy it.
- I used to enjoy it.
- To be reassured that I am loved.
- To reconnect when we have resolved a problem between us.
- To communicate with my partner.
- To celebrate my masculinity/femininity.
- For intimacy.
- To share my joy.
- I desire to share love with my partner.
- I feel loved.
- We have some quality time on our own.
- Sex connects us deeply.
- During sex I forget the rest of the world.
  ....
  ....
  ....(your own reasons).

These questions can help you to consider what you think are positive and negative reasons for sex.

Return to the list and ask the title question a slightly different way:

What reasons would you choose for having sex?

Write these answers on a separate piece of paper. Again, answer 'Yes' or 'No' against each question. Compare your two sets of answers.

- Did you feel unsure how to answer any of the questions?
- Did you feel anxious when you read any of the questions?
- Were your two sets of answers different?
- Were more questions sparked in your mind?

If you were unsure, anxious or the two sets of answers were different – then you might like to make some changes in your sexual life. If you are uncertain as to what changes and how to make them, you will find the rest of the book guides you through your concerns.

When you reach the end of the book do return to this questionnaire. You may find that some of your answers are different.

∽

Is it lust or love?

*Sugar and spice and all things nice
That's what little girls are made of.
Slugs and snails and puppy dogs tails
That's what little boys are made of.*

Nursery rhyme

Chapter Two

Boy meets girl

*E*yes meet (was it really across a crowded room?), sparks fly and courtship begins. If all is going well, being together in some established way seems promising. A voyage begins to look interesting. But is he dreaming of an action-packed adventure while she muses on the prospect of romantic interludes under the stars?

How can a man and woman be mates aboard the love boat? Are men and women incomprehensible to each other? Are men only interested in sex? Are women only interested in intimate talks? We have said 'Yes' to such questions through the ages. But where does it take us on the voyage to discover happiness between men and women?

John Gray in his popular book *Men are from Mars, Women are from Venus*, reinforced what you already knew. Men and women are different. This simplistic view does little to help you understand differences and respect each other as equals. Subscription to this self-limiting prejudice results in the belief that men and women can never understand each other. For harmony you need to overcome such prejudice, not reinforce it.

I heard more enlightening information on Venus and Mars, surprisingly, during an ABC television programme on astronomy.

'Venus, Mars and Earth have the same source of planetary mass. Planetary probes revealed startling differences and remarkable similarities.'

What are the 'startling differences and remarkable similarities' between men and women in sexual relationships? It is easy to recognise the differences. They dangle in front of you! But the physically obvious can make you overlook the similarities. Men and women are not the same, although both are human. Both desire sexual relationships, want them to work, want to feel close and want to feel fulfilled. The popularity of marriage affirms these common goals. The path of a man may, however, be different to a woman in achieving these goals.

If you are willing to look at both sides as having value, gender differences cease to be a trial of right and wrong. Instead, they become interesting and present opportunities to expand your beliefs .

Biological difference

There are some inherited differences in the way that males and females behave. We are learning in non-sexual areas to understand these differences. As a result change is being achieved that was previously thought to be impossible.

Girls, for example, learn to read more quickly than boys. This language skill related to the sense of hearing comes more naturally to girls. It is an inborn gender difference. We know that boys find visual concepts easier than girls. Some clever researchers have taught boys to read just as quickly as girls by showing them pictures of lip movements for each sound. Explained to boys on their own wavelength, boys learn to read as fast as girls.

Is sexuality the final frontier to be explored to achieve understanding between men and women? Can you learn to tune in on his/her sex wavelength? We know men have more testosterone than women. This is a startling difference. One result may be a higher inborn drive for sex in men. Sexual drive supports a reproductive necessity ensuring his genes are passed on to the next generation. If you accept this biological imperative, it makes sense of research findings that really come as no surprise. Men rate fertility signals in women: breasts, hips and youth, high on the attraction scale.

Women may have a higher inborn desire for a long-term mate. Desire may be nature's way to ensure that the genes from the woman survive due to the care that can be offered children in an ongoing relationship. This makes sense of the results of the other part of the research. Women rate commitment signals: sensitive eyes, good job, attention to her, high on the attraction scale. Hairy chests, muscles, big penises seldom get a rating.[2]

Not only is testosterone a factor in sexual drive but it is also associated with aggressive behaviour. This may contribute to men acting in 'macho' ways that seem very different and incomprehensible to women. In the cave men era these behaviours were essential to survival. One million years later our basic drives are modified by the additional brainpower of thinking. Now both male and female are wanting more than reproductive success in relationships. We yearn for the advanced human experience of happiness. Inherited behaviours, suited only to reproduction and survival of the fittest, are insufficient for love and intimacy.

We are changing how we act towards each other. To move beyond our cavemen ancestors, men and women are learning to appreciate the different values of drive and desire, but it requires a stretch of the mind for both. Being open to reconsider your views is the very essence of embracing the differences between men and women for mutual benefit and sexual fulfilment. There is more on this theme later in *The Voyage of Love & Sex*.

Roles assigned by gender

Another startling biological difference is that women bear children and men cannot. In the past this resulted in a clear definition between male and female roles in society. Men were the providers and held powerful positions in the community. Women were homemakers and raised children. These exclusive roles had limitations. They have now gone past their 'use by' date.

The advantages in the past for a woman in her rigid role were shrouded in the romantic 'in love' myth. A knight in shining armour would sweep her off her feet. He would provide for her and make her happy for the rest of their life.

The 'knight' would expect to come home to a cooked meal, children bathed and in bed, and dictate what he wanted, including sexually. Supposedly this should delight his wife. But the 'damsel' ended up doing things she often did not enjoy. As a wife she had no financial independence and was unable to explore her full potential. The husband was also limited by his rigid role. He had to work for the rest of his life to provide for his family, often in a job that was soul destroying.

Of course, gender roles are changing. Change is an inevitable part of life but it is not an easy process. Both men and women, trying to chart their changing course, have ended up struggling with extra demands at work and home. Both feel the economic pressures of our modern world. A large number of women now pursue their own careers. However, statistics show that working women are still doing more domestic work than their working husbands. Women are seeking the recognition of equal sharing in daily workload both paid and unpaid as roles become less defined.

I explored this topic when speaking at a 'Women in the Workforce' conference.

I asked the audience, "How many of your partners are delighted you go to work?" Several hands were raised. Then I asked, "Leave your hands up if your partner automatically does a fair share of housework." Only two hands remained. The other women were laughing at the question.

It seems that working men and women have not yet been successful in resolving this problem in a way that is respectful to both. This art of respectful discussion and then doing what has been agreed upon is a much-neglected art of which you can read more in Chapter Twelve. It has significance in a harmonious relationship, beyond the specific topic of household chores. You may wonder what is the relevance of the seemingly unimportant subject of housework to sexual relationships. But unfairness based on assumption of gender difference is one of the commonest problems to be raised by couples in distress. Any problem that causes distress eventually finds its way into the bedroom.

Fair sharing of tasks of any sort is symbolic of equality and respect. It does not mean doing half of every individual chore but working out a system that feels equal to both. Individuals can be respected for their individual skills, ability and personal inclination. There will be gender differences. They need to be understood and discussed for mutual understanding. Then a team is formed which can function better than either individual. For the team to function well the rules can no longer be based on gender assumptions.

Problem solving

Men and women have often developed a different approach to problems. For women it is common that talking and sharing of feelings are part of female upbringing. For men it is action, the doing, that is the shared male learning experience. What can be the benefit of valuing the differences as equal?

Jim, the father of Daniel (aged 7) and Melissa (aged 9) explained how he noticed the gender differences in his own children, which made him consider this question.

"Melissa was playing netball at school. She fell and cut her leg. She burst into tears and hobbled off the netball court. Within a few moments the rest of her team followed her. Between them they washed Melissa's knee, comforted her, sympathised with her pain, bandaged her knee and together they returned to continue the game," Jim said.

"On another occasion Daniel was playing football. He was running so hard that he fell. The game continued. The others ran past him as he picked himself up. He fixed his eye on the ball rolling past him and in spite of the pain in his knee he ran forward. With all his might and with extra energy he scored a goal. The rest of the team congratulated Daniel for his bravery. I was proud of him and stood on the sidelines cheering him on. The difference between girls and boys really struck me," Jim pondered.

"Melissa's knee was better in a few days but Daniel needed to see a physiotherapist for treatment. As I sat in the physio's waiting room, I thought Daniel might have been better off if he had stopped for a while. Melissa's team lost their match. I wondered if they would have had a better chance of winning if Melissa had gone off the court alone to have her knee fixed. It seemed to me they could each learn from each other," Jim mused.

You may think that the different ways men and women solve problems confirms they are born on different planets. But how much is inborn nature, and how much is a result of learning? Scientists are still arguing the toss between nature and nurture. Rather than assume an irreconcilable difference it is helpful to think in terms of feminine and masculine styles.

Greg and Pauline (whom you will meet in greater depth in Chapter Nine) illustrate this difference.

"Monty, our Labrador, had been run over. He was lying on the road, whimpering. I wanted Greg to hold me, to understand how upset I felt. Any one of my girlfriends would have hugged me automatically. He is such a block he didn't," Pauline complained.

"I was just as upset but I had to do something. My mate next door was a real help. He picked up Monty, put him in the car and took the dog to the vet. He joked on the way and that helped to relieve the emotion for me. Pauline was wailing in the back of the car. I told her not to upset herself, but she kept on crying." Greg shrugged his shoulders.

You may detect that Greg thinks Pauline's way is wrong and she thinks he is wrong. Greg and Pauline were both upset, but expressed their distress differently. The support they each preferred was also different.

A couple can struggle with their differences or place their effort into understanding each other.

When a woman has a problem she wants her partner to listen, to attempt to understand, and offer support without immediately providing practical solutions. A man may seek a different style of support. He may require practical suggestions and practical help. Yet somewhere inside Greg was a part that would have found relief in sobbing about his dog. Somewhere inside Pauline a practical response was lurking. I asked how each would have handled the situation on their own.

"Of course I would have got the dog to the vet if I'd been the only one there." Pauline sat straight upright in her full dignity.

"I would have put Monty in the car. I suppose I might have had a few tears on the way to the vet. Monty was really hurt." Greg softened momentarily.

Do you accept traditional gender differences as absolute or do you acknowledge the value in both?

Styles of intimacy

Men are often accused of thinking of nothing but sex, as though they are obsessed with the physical act. Yet when I listen to men I hear that sex is not only physical it is an important expression of intimacy for them. Male culture gives the OK to intimacy in the disguise of sex. Men may not have ways to discuss loving emotion with their father or friends but sex is their opportunity. However, they may need to adopt 'macho' attitudes to express themselves with other men. Sex talk of conquests and performances is shared but talk about intimacy is not. To admit to a problem with sex is even more difficult. He runs the risk of being seen as less manly than others.

Women base their intimacy on talking with one another. Emotional support from female friends is the result. Talking intimacy has the stamp of approval of female culture. Sex talk linked to the emotion of love is shared. Sex talk of conquests and performance is more limited.

These different approaches to intimacy can lead to great misunderstanding particularly if each insists that their way is the only true intimacy. How does it feel for men to open to talking intimacy? How does it feel for women to open to sexual intimacy? Later in the book couples face these very questions.

Underlying these styles is a double standard of sexual conduct. There are centuries of belief that men could 'sow their wild oats' but 'nice girls don't'. If you think this view is out of date you will be surprised by a 1992 survey[3] of 15 to 17-year-old Australians (male and female). The majority described boys favourably as 'studs' if they had casual sex. Girls doing the same thing were put down as 'sluts'.

These same adolescents thought boys could not control their sexual urges but girls could. Such thinking removes personal responsibility for behaviour with the excuse of being 'born that way and I can't help myself'. We have abandoned this particular line of thought in other areas such as crime. Could we also relegate this to the past in sexual behaviour?

Understanding and appreciating difference
Of course, men and women are different but that does not mean you cannot be on the same team, enjoying the benefits of sharing your different values. A relationship can allow a man the opportunity to experience 'feminine' ways and a woman to experience 'masculine' ways. This is quite different from the romantic notion of finding your other half. Then logically two half people make a total of one. An intimate relationship can stimulate you to become complete within your self and combine to make a total of two.

Romantic tales do not help you to do this. You do not learn these lessons at school. Unfortunately, you rarely learn this from your parents. They were shaped from a different culture less questioning of ideas fixed in gender but their approach did not lead them to discover the secret of happiness in relationships. Will equality and respect bring this? I feel it has a better chance of doing so.

Perhaps you and your partner have already learned to resolve differences in a way that enriches you. If you have not then this book helps you through that process. To reach a solution that is respectful of both, differences need to be heard and understood.

For all the theories of gender difference, the important issue is the individuality of your self and your partner, whatever gender you may be. Not only may you be of different gender but each has grown up in a unique family with different values. You bring to your love relationship a wealth of separate experiences from childhood, through teenage years into adulthood.

You will have areas of similarity, perhaps common interests or common goals that brought you together. Yet there are always differences. You can dismiss them as incomprehensible, blaming gender alone, or with effort appreciate their value and learn from each other.

We accept and expect progress in other spheres such as technology, medicine and sport. Then why not progress in sexual relationships? They certainly require similar effort if we want to reach our full potential. Sticking with the caveman philosophy of 'me man, you woman' is limited and results in much distress. Women, when they want to be, can be just as passionate as men. Men can choose to be just as thoughtful and nurturing as women. It takes courage to break free of gender stereotypes. This effort is the path to peace between people who are different.

You will need a willingness to let go of fixed ideas that one gender is right, the other wrong. If you limit your self in this way the best you can achieve is to tolerate your partner by adopting a patronising attitude. Would you really be satisfied long term with such banal suggestions as a man saying, "I'll give you long slow sex whenever you want (which I don't think is very often) if you give me a 'quickie' whenever I want." Or a woman saying, "You help me with the housework (which I don't think will be very often) and I'll feel more like having sex with you." This does nothing to address the underlying problems though it may stick a band-aid over them. But eventually goodwill is eroded and happiness may be destroyed by temporary measures.

Imagine the strengths of a sexual relationship where the man knows and understands his sensual pleasures and has opened to his feelings and those of his partner. Imagine the joy of the female who knows her feelings and has opened to her sensual pleasure and that of her partner. This would be drive and desire blended for mutual benefit. If you can fully respect difference and expand to explore the potential benefits of both you can have it all.

Treating each individual as different and equal is essential in all relationships not just sexual ones. Men or women, old or young, black or white, Jew or Moslem are all worthy of understanding. We have the capacity to review our differences, understand each other and make some shifts in thinking. This skill of thinking beyond your own way is essential in the discussion of differences. The 'how to' is explained in Chapter Twelve.

"Unto the woman," He said,
"I will greatly multiply thy sorrow and thy conception;
In sorrow thou shalt bring forth children."

Genesis 3:6. Old Testament

Chapter Three

Who makes the rules?

Before you are allowed to embark on the love boat you have to learn the rules that apply aboard. But who makes these rules and how did he get to be captain? If sex combines a basic drive essential for reproduction with personal desire, why have so many regulations sprung up to control this natural process?

How did the amazing kaleidoscope of beliefs, morals and taboos come about?

Family, friends and teachers supplied brochures packed with their own views about shipboard rules. Then of course, culture, religion and community had something to add. Radio, television, international travel and the Internet has expanded your thinking to include global ideas. As a social being influenced by the ideas of others, some will suit your voyage well; others will be at odds with what you believe deep inside your self.

When you take the time to identify the source of your beliefs, you may realise that some of what you hold true is really a truth for Mum, Dad, a teacher, media, or a religion. Your mature adult self needs to sift through beliefs formed in the past and decide which are really right for you at this moment.

Culture and religion in the past

Present day beliefs are still underpinned by centuries of sexual rules and regulations. A glimpse at the history of sexual beliefs is fascinating. The weird, the wonderful, the puritanical, the bizarre – we have tried it all. Yet society is still unsettled with sexuality. Governments, religions, medics and fortune seekers have offered rules, promises and potions to regulate our sexuality. Somewhere between the extremes of public orgies and enforced celibacy you can arrive at your own balance. At last there is the freedom to choose your own way to be comfortable with sexuality.

The history of sex in society reveals some clues as to why many are still struggling to find their sexual harmony. In ancient times views were very different from today. Voluptuous replicas of goddesses have been found in the ruins of many civilisations. Females were seen to emanate a life-producing force as demonstrated by their ability to bear children. Goddesses were worshipped for their power in the natural world. Was this pagan ignorance or ancient wisdom?

Why did it all change? The Judaeo/Christian religion introduced an all-powerful male god replacing the female as creator. In the process celebration of female sexuality was seen as uncivilised and sinful. The first female in the Bible, Eve, was cursed for seducing Adam, hardly an encouraging start for women or men to find joy in sexuality.

Towards the end of the Greek-Roman era the disapproval of pleasure, particularly sexual pleasure, was promoted by the philosophers of the day. At the same time, Emperor Constantine decreed Christianity to be the official religion of the Roman world.

No longer were there goddesses of sexuality and fertility. Their image could not be destroyed altogether but was altered to re-emerge in the shape of the Virgin Mary. This version of female deity represented a major divergence from the sexuality of previous goddesses. Now the conception of a child of God occurred without sexual intercourse. The worship of Chastity began.

The celebration of women's sexuality was replaced by guilt and sin fitting neatly within the patriarchy that the Judeao/Christian religion had created. Men had taken control of women's sexuality and it became the property of men. But trying to control others comes at a price. Early monks had to face the dilemma presented by their views on sex. Chastity was seen as pure and spiritual yet they were troubled by normal human sexual desire. To reach spiritual fulfilment they struggled to suppress their sexual feelings and expected others to do the same. The tyranny of the Church rather than the charitable spirit of the religious texts took control of sexuality.

St. Augustine (AD 354-430) has much to answer for. He and his order of monks promoted the view that sexuality was base and to be controlled if not extinguished. Lust was a sin. Sex even for reproduction was barely tolerated. Other aspects of sexuality such as desire, expression of love, masturbation, erotica and sexual pleasure were considered appalling and the work of the devil.

The mood of sexual repression persisted through the centuries. You may smile as you read a proclamation by the Archbishop of Canterbury from the Penitence list compiled in 8th century England. Seven year's penitence was declared a suitable time to atone for committing premeditated murder. The sin of oral sex however, demanded up to a lifetime of penitence. Sex was more likely to lead to purgatory than murder.

Church leaders in the 13th century, for instance, declared that rear entry sex was permitted only in certain medical conditions but even then could only be indulged in if it were done with 'a pain in the soul'. Such ideas must have created a quandary for people of the time who knew their own natural desires but were told by the church that they were wrong. It is a predicament many still face in the world today.

Since ordinary people were not thought to be able to communicate with God directly the Church acted as intermediary thereby being able to set out all the rules for living. The serfs of the feudal system were to have no power, particularly from a divine source. The clergy maintained their elevated position by chanting to God in Latin, a language mysterious to common folk. The translation of the Bible into English and its printing in the 16th century enormously increased access to the word of God. The monopoly of knowledge by the established Church began to be challenged.

The emergence of science in the Renaissance led to heated debate between the clergy and scientists regarding research using dissection of the human bodies. Eventually a deal was struck between the powerful groups. The spirit was assigned to the clergy, the body to doctors and the mind to philosophers. This fatal separation was to limit care for the whole person for 500 years in the West.

Some Eastern religions did not suffer from this theological tussle. Instead the joy of human sex was celebrated in their religious ideology. Their places of worship have been adorned throughout the ages with representation of male and female genitals carved in stone. This is not in worship of promiscuity but in recognition of the strength of sex in loving relationships. Hindus and Buddhists consider it possible to transcend to an awareness of self within the universe, as a connection with the divine. Sexual communion is considered one of the ways to achieve this. These religions consider chastity of their monks as simply a different spiritual path.

But Western culture in the past did not entertain this view of sex. English ladies and gentlemen in India during the British Raj, glimpsing sexually explicit carvings in temples, were apparently shocked, their sensibilities offended. Swooning, or at least an embarrassed blush, were suitable responses. Yet in the ultimate hypocrisy scandalous affairs, bordellos and syphilis thrived at the same time.

Suppression of sexual joy was in full force in the Victorian era. Dr. J. H. Kellogg of Kellogg's Corn Flakes fame wrote a best selling book in 1888 which contained horrifying 'facts' on the evils of sexuality. He instructed parents to be vigilant for the signs of masturbation in their children. He listed 33 such signs including rounded shoulders, acne and epilepsy. He even invented several contraptions to prevent children touching their genitals in bed at night. A lockable metal cage to cover the pelvic area was one of his designs for this purpose. His huge success with Corn Flakes was due to their promotion as an anti-masturbatory food. It was not necessary to provide evidence for such claims in that era.

Here again we have an 'authority' telling people how to behave sexually. Sexuality was regulated without compassion. Homosexuality was decreed a criminal offence and remained so until recent years. Difference was feared rather than understood.

Marriage manuals of the Victorian era recommended that a loving husband would perform his marital sex as quickly as possible so as not to upset his wife who, being female, would not enjoy intercourse. In contrast there was the reality of a large number of prostitutes catering for the 'animal' instincts of men.

We can understand why people would turn to higher authorities for sexual guidance at this time. The world was facing the horrors of the sexually transmitted disease – syphilis. This disease led to severe heart damage, insanity and eventually death. The ravages of syphilis did not occur so long ago; some grandparents can still remember the time before antibiotics were available to treat the disease.

The American response led to the foundation of the Young Men's Christian Association (YMCA). The aim was to distract young men from wasting their energy in sexual pursuits by substituting all male sporting activity thereby saving young men from syphilis. Instead their young bodies were prepared for the more 'suitable' pursuit of fighting in the First World War.

Two World Wars brought great changes in thinking. Young people became aware of death in the present. Many traditional ideas were challenged, including sexual morality. Books on contraception began to appear amidst public outcry. Families unable to raise large numbers of children privately welcomed them. People knew that high pregnancy rates and poverty had contributed to frighteningly high death rates in mothers and newborn babies. The opportunity to reduce family size without abstaining from sex was very attractive. At last it was possible to separate the pleasure of sexual intercourse from the consequence of babies.

The role of women too was changing. They gained the vote and joined the workforce, which led to a level of independence. The time of peace that followed the World Wars was also a time of economic growth. Money became available for medical research. As a result the 'Pill', the next step in liberating men and women to explore their sexual potential, hit the world in the 1960s. This was the era of 'free love' with the slogan, 'make love, not war'. The 'flower people' hoped that free love would bring peace and happiness. But many found that free love did not fulfil their dreams of peace, happiness or sexual joy. They found that more was not necessarily better. They knew much more about how to do 'it' and how to have sex without getting pregnant, but still that was not enough. The body had been liberated but not the mind.

In the early 1980s a new disease, AIDS, entered the sexual arena. It is caused by a virus, HIV, which can be sexually transmitted. This life threatening disease is spreading throughout the world; the poorer the community the greater the devastation. It has become even more imperative to have full knowledge to make your own decisions about sexual behaviour.

We can move beyond the authoritarian dictates on sexuality of the past. Yet as some strive to evolve in sexual awareness there are still examples of repression in the world today. In Africa and areas of the Middle East genital mutilation of female children, often without anaesthetic, is still being performed. This extreme practice veiled in cultural and religious dogma aims to remove sexual sensation, in women. 130 million women in the world today have been abused in this way.

They took everything that God gave me to enjoy being a woman.
Waris Dirie, supermodel born in Somalia

It appears respect for individual sexual choice has some way to go in our world.

Your choice in the present

The early era of the baby boomers was a materialistic one – the focus for happiness was external, often embodied in the accumulation of material goods. In Western culture this perpetuated the belief that happiness would be obtained through winning the State lottery. Yet happiness dependent on wealth from outside your self appears to be, at best, short-lived. Given an increasingly long life span you may be looking for a more sustainable source of happiness. The focus is now shifting to an inner source of happiness. Relationships, sexuality and self esteem are being more valued in this regard.

Life crises spotlight attention on finding a balance between exterior demands and inner desires. The troubled times in your sexual relationship are common crises. Beliefs rooted in the past come under review. The commitment to soulless striving, to benefit others but not your self, is being reassessed in work and in personal life.

Not only baby boomers, but also increasing numbers of younger people, are facing the same predicament. Perhaps with the uncertainty of the economic future the emphasis on an external source to provide happiness is being questioned earlier in life.

One of the essential ingredients of inner peace is a personal ease with your sexual hopes, dreams and desires. The centuries of religious dogma that viewed sexual pleasure as sinful were shed with a pendulum swing to a belief that more sex with more people was pleasure. The fulfilment of human sexual potential lies in finding your own balance between these extremes, one that brings a sexual connection respectful of your self and your partner.

Who makes the rules?

I learned that it always makes me feel good to see my parents holding hands.

'Age 13'
Live, Learn and Pass It On
H. Jackson Brown, Jr

Chapter Four
Lessons and teachers

If you plan to spend your life on a voyage it can be life saving to know how to swim, to sail, to navigate, and have a sense of direction. Over the years of childhood did your teachers make sure you learned all these skills before setting sail?

In Western culture the aim of education is to help a child become knowledgeable and therefore independent. Much time is spent coming to grips with reading, writing and arithmetic in school and perhaps college or university, to gain more knowledge. Yet what did you learn as a child that prepared you for the adult world of sexual relationships, that would have far more impact on your life than the three 'R's?

You may have had a hotch-potch of experience before any specific sex education began. Sniggering behind the bike sheds, paying a few cents to see the mystery lying hidden under a pair of knickers, trying furtive kisses, watching television or reading romantic novels provided an unreliable basis for approaching a relationship. A more sinister influence has crept in via movies and computer games in which violence is portrayed as the way to get what you want.

Who provided guidance to help you develop happiness in a relationship of love and sex? Schools and families generally supply the basic facts about body function. But sex education often ignores the roller coaster of feelings, thoughts, lustiness, desires and hopes that are the context of personal relationships.

Family

Your education began with watching the way Mum and Dad treated each other. At home was there warmth or conflict between Mum and Dad, between you and them? As you began to ask questions, were they open and honest about sexuality? Was there careful explanation appropriate to your age? Or were your parents awkward about love and sex? Was sex a taboo subject?

It is not easy for adults to take up the challenge that a new generation presents, with their sexual curiosity. Considering the history of sexual repression in our culture this is not surprising. No where are there more half-truths told than in sexuality. Tales of storks, cabbage patches eggs and seeds abound.

What words did you learn to describe parts of your body? You probably heard the correct word for other parts of the body - nose, arms and eyes. But what were you told to call a penis - willy, dick, winkle, old fella? There are many more. What about vagina - down below, between the legs, even middle bottom? Some girls have no word at all. With nothing obvious to point or hold on to it is possible for a girl to ignore this vital part of her body for years.

Worse, these are the parts of the body degraded to swear words - cunt, dickhead, prick. These are harsh words that represent a general disgust with genitals, which is sad considering their delightful role in sexual pleasure.

It is not only what adults said but also what they did that affected your learning process. You will have received many messages about communication, intimacy and sexuality from your parent's behaviour.

Both you and they may have been completely unaware of the subtle transfer of information.

Positive learning

Did you see your parents openly kiss and cuddle, not only each other but you as well? They were sending positive messages about affectionate touch. Respectful touch is an essential reinforcement of love for a child. Lost, hurt or unsure, a hug can make all the difference.

Did your parents honour their own private area in the house? Did they make a rule that you had to knock before entering their bedroom? Did you hear happy sounds coming out of their bedroom? Did they in turn respect your own space? Privacy helps you develop as separate members of a family.

Was each family member given time to talk about their concerns, to understand and respect each other even when you did not agree? Did Mum and Dad solve problems in mutual respect? These send positive signals about the value of individual difference.

Was there a blend of praise and caution that contributed to your sense of well being? Did you understand why Mum and Dad wanted to know where you were and who with? These can be acts of love and concern.

You may not have thought of these behaviours as being part of sex education but they concern honesty, love, touch, respect of private time and individual views, problem solving and self esteem – the basics of relationship.

In addition, to integrate sexuality into your life, the related body functions – erections, wet dreams, menstruation, sexual intercourse and pregnancy need to be talked about as normal. When discussed without shame, without fear or exaggeration, they are an essential part of preparation for the voyage. Ignorance is not bliss.

A friend told a delightful example of a positive message to me. It concerned her five-year-old son, Ben. She had read a fairy story to him called, *The King Who Liked Bouncing*. This was her shortened version:

> *The elderly king died leaving his young son to be king. The boy loved to bounce on any thing soft. But once he was king his advisors told him to stop, as it wasn't correct behaviour for a king. The king became sad and then very ill. His advisors were so worried they asked if there was anything that would make the little king feel better. He replied that he would like to be allowed to bounce whenever he wanted. They all agreed. The king bounced up and down on his bed. He was so happy. His advisors were also happy. They joined in and found out that they enjoyed bouncing too.*

At the end of the story Ben made a knowing statement:
"So that's why you and Daddy bounce up and down on the bed with no clothes on. Is it fun for you?"
"Yes, it certainly is. We call it sex," His mother wisely replied.

She had sent a positive message about sex to her 5-year-old son and took the opportunity to offer more by asking if he wanted to know anything else about sex. She answered all his questions in full honesty.

It would be wonderful to receive only positive lessons from your family. But as perfect parents are unknown it is likely you also picked up some negative attitudes.

Negative learning

Did your mother or father shriek and grab a towel when you innocently walked into the bathroom when he/she was naked? This response sends a clear message that there is something wrong with nakedness.

As you explored your own body and alighted on self pleasure when you touched your clitoris or penis, did you hear, "Don't do that it's naughty," or even get a smack. Was there any explanation given? Later in adolescent years when you self pleasured (masturbated) did you feel a tinge of guilt? Were you worried that an adult might catch you out? Through these lessons you learn to associate the unpleasant feeling of guilt with sexuality.

This negativity is compounded by the untruths that some parents tell to cover their embarrassment at a sexual question. It is amazing that in this very important area of our lives some adults still avoid being honest. A promise to tell more 'when you are old enough to understand', sends a message that the truth may be unpleasant or the child was wrong to even ask. Of course it does nothing to quell the curiosity of a child who will merely look for another, often less reliable, source. Children are always old enough to understand the truth.

Girls learn about periods, period pain, vaginal discharges, pregnancy, almost as a price for womanhood. The joys of sexuality are often missing from this introduction to maturity. Is this our pleasureless legacy of religious views on sex and sin? In some cultures, however, the onset of puberty is celebrated in young women. Would it be beneficial if we developed a rite of passage appropriate to our own culture?

Boys too may blush with the embarrassment of puberty. Friends tease when a boy has an erection. A first wet dream may be heralded by sheets being bundled up and furtively thrown into the laundry. This new world of sexual awareness can be full of uncertainty, sometimes the honest and understanding words, which can demystify this awakening, remain unsaid.

What was communication like in your home? Was there a hostile atmosphere – endless arguments, sulking, days of no communication, intimidation or even violence? Did the members of your family put each other down? If you learn that messages between male and female are all about power and control then sexual connection occurs on the same wavelength.

As you read these questions and recall your own experiences you realise the impact of parents on your own attitudes towards love and sex. You may have moved beyond the standards of your parents but this early learning leaves a lasting impression. Parents cannot teach more than they know. If they have a screwed up personal life, you see it all. You can accept or reject what they offer. Either way they leave their mark. Later in life you may decide to review what you learned in your family and decide on any change in your thinking and behaviour that would allow you to feel happier in your own relationships.

School

Some teachers struggle with sex education finding it difficult to provide a balance between information, caution and celebration. Did your school do this well? The basic workings of reproduction were often the starting point for sex education. The risks of sex were usually covered – pregnancy, abortion, sexually transmitted diseases, AIDS. Did this scare the life out of you or did your teachers find a way to balance the problems with the joys? If you learned these basics did you also know what to do about your sex drive? Did you learn how to handle a 'crush', your first love, intimacy, wanting someone so much you could not sleep or did you have to work that out on your own?

Unfortunately, many teachers are themselves unskilled in this area. The education system still leaves the decision to include sexual relationships in the curriculum to a matter of choice. It is strange to me that it should be treated so differently from any other subject.

In the United States there are movements to reduce the range of information even further. The 'True Love Waits' campaign promotes abstinence as a method of reducing unwanted pregnancies and the incidence of AIDS. It is likely to be as successful as prohibition of alcohol was in that same country!

More, not less, knowledge in essential life skills allows you to make your own informed decisions. As a child gradually discovers sexuality it is important that parents and teachers provide appropriate information. A balance between privacy and exposure, safety and risk are essential for a child to become fully aware. From this awareness develops the confidence to know what you feel comfortable with and what feels uncomfortable. The respect of your own body and sexuality is a precious learning to be gained from adults.

Self Exploration

You, of course, learned much for your self from your own inquisitiveness. You probably played games of 'doctors and nurses'. Ronald and Juliette Goldman in their book, *Show Me Yours*,[4] which researched sexuality in the U.S.A., Australia, England and Sweden, showed that 83% of children explored their genitals either alone or with a similar aged friend. It was, however, often concealed and associated with a feeling of doing something wrong. Yet this is normal healthy exploration.

Children brought up in the country see animals mating and learn the mechanics of intercourse. Plenty of children also sneak a look at human lovers to satisfy their curiosity though they may not always make sense of what they see and hear.

Parents are often disturbed about the good and bad of touch. In our culture there is less touch than in some others and obviously this varies between families. If you were brought up in a family where there was little touch you may feel neglected in this area. Alternatively you may feel too much touch intruded into your personal space. How much is right for a child? Enough makes you feel loved, wanted and respected.

It has a quality that encourages you to reach out at any age and touch when you want to feel the presence of another.

Both parents and children may be confused about what is the wrong kind of touch. This can be particularly difficult for fathers with their daughters when there is now much attention given to incest. But there is an obvious difference between an affectionate cuddle that respects the integrity of the child and abusive touch, for the benefit of the adult. It is sad if a child misses out on affectionate touch because adults are unsure about correct behaviour. Touch respectful of the child can be the gentlest connection and a reassuring sign of love.

Sexual abuse

Consenting sexual play between children or respectful touch by an adult is not to be confused with the unwanted intrusion by another (often older) person. If a child is somehow involved in the sexual activity of an older person that is sexual abuse. It is thought that one in four female children and perhaps one in eight male children have experienced intrusion into their private sexual integrity. The effects on the child in their growing sexuality is always negative. The extent of the damage depends on many other learning processes occurring at the time.

In a family where there is openness, equality, stability, where the child can talk to an adult, be believed and have appropriate action taken, the damage can be significantly diminished. In a family where there are secrets, where there is intimidation, abuse – verbal, physical or sexual – then it is extremely difficult for the child to be heard, believed and for the abuse to cease.

> *All is well in the family. This isn't really happening. Ignore it and it goes away. Their reaction takes me deeper into my emotions as I remember*

this scene happening so many times before. How does incest survive in a family?

This is how it survives – by backs being turned and ears being shut.

'Feeling is Healing'[5]
Women's Project Group, Qld

Very few people exit a family with a strong self-esteem and for those with the added wound of sexual abuse, living fully can be a considerable challenge.

If you have been sexually abused in childhood and you wish to discuss this, a professional experienced in the field of sexual abuse can be very helpful. The aim of such counselling should not be to revisit the past relentlessly but to assist you to develop your full potential in the present. This development is very much the substance of the following chapters in this book. You will find these ideas helpful though they are not specifically directed at people who have been sexually abused. They do tackle many elements of difficult learning from childhood to enable you to move beyond surviving to thriving.

Reaching your potential

We expect to receive Grade 'A' for achievement in Love, Sex, Intimacy and Relationships. But unfortunately our groundwork is shaky and lessons are often inadequate, distorted or absent. How do you reach a high standard as an adult? You can try some adult education. You will need to be willing to strive for a gold star for effort. But these subjects are worth every bit of effort you make, not just a short burst but with commitment to a continuing process. It takes time to review early lessons and practice to make updates and persist with change. As you reconsider your childhood learning you and your sexual relationship can grow to meet your dreams. (Chapter Eleven takes this topic further.)

But first you need to decide on what you want to focus your attention. This questionnaire allows you to consider what you knew before your first sexual experience. Ideally this information is accumulated over many years provided prior to being needed but often is not. Were you as well informed as you would have like to be? Are your children (if you have any) better informed? What lessons did you miss?

What did you learn before your first sexual experience?

	Everything	Fair bit	Not much	Nothing much
Facts				
name of genitals				
masturbation				
body changes with age				
sex drive				
periods				
erections				
ejaculation				
sexual intercourse				
hormones				
pregnancy				
sexual difficulties				
problems for disabled				
sexual abuse				
sexual violence				
STD				
HIV/AIDS				
Emotions				
falling in love				
sexual attraction				
changes in long-term relationships				
sexual desire				
sexual preferences				
intimacy				
affairs				

	Everything	Fair bit	Not much	Nothing much

Self Respect
peer pressure
confidence
respectful behaviour
listening to your Self
self esteem
respectful discussion
  of difference

Are there any topics in this list that you want to attend to now? Since your first sexual experience you will have learned much more about love and sex and will continue to do so as life and love present you with the unexpected. The course of this voyage unfolds in the next part of the book.

∼

*You ought not to attempt to cure the . . .
body without the soul;
and this is the reason why the cure of
many diseases is unknown
to the physicians of Hellas,
because they are ignorant of the whole,
. . . for the part can never be well unless the whole is well.*

'Charmides'
Plato

Chapter Five

Only flesh and blood?

Would you call the ship's doctor when the love boat hits a storm or are the captain and crew more important in keeping you on course? Perhaps they all need to be consulted for the best chance to stay afloat.

Your sexual health is dependent on many factors but do you think of your self as made of only flesh and blood? If you do, you may be concerned by the implication of the mind in a sexual problem. This may suggest to you that the problem is only a figment of your imagination and has no reality. Yet physical and mental processes are intricately linked.

Western medicine is now understanding the impact that one has on the other. Scientific studies have clearly shown the links between stress and health problems such as heart attacks, digestion problems, and alcohol abuse – the list is enormous. Chemical deficiencies have been found in the brain in illnesses such as depression previously labelled as 'mental'.

The workings of the mind affect the health of the body and vice versa. Both body and mind are important in sexuality.

There are of course some physical problems that overwhelm sexual function. The spirit may be willing but the body is weak. When the spirit is truly willing much sexual pleasure can still be enjoyed, even by those with considerable physical problems. In fact, some people embrace their physical difficulties to gain a fresh perspective on life. In doing so their sexual intimacy can be enhanced. Physical limitations can challenge some to achieve a level of sexual intimacy of which more able-bodied people may only dream.

A few years ago I was speaking at a conference on arthritis. A young woman, Jackie, told me of the unusual severity of her rheumatoid arthritis. Many of her joints were clearly misshapen. She explained that sometimes her joints were so stiff that even simple movements became impossible. Jackie had been married for five years but she had had her arthritis since she was a young girl. She introduced me to her husband, Paul, then continued.

"I wanted to tell you about our sex. Since we first married my hips have become worse. Sometimes when I wanted to have sex with Paul my hips are too stiff and painful. It used to make me feel so sad. Sometimes I'd fancy him like crazy and I couldn't do anything."

Paul smiled and explained reassuringly, *"I knew Jackie could be uncomfortable because of her arthritis but also feel sexy. The fact that intercourse wasn't always possible was no big issue for me. I'm happy to caress Jackie. I love to see her get turned on."*

"I felt a bit strange at first not being able to do the real thing," said Jackie. *"But what Paul did felt so beautiful, I found myself becoming comfortable to caress him too. We both become aroused and reach orgasm even when intercourse isn't possible."*

There was such gentleness and understanding for each other as they described their sexual intimacy. Whispering so only Paul and I could hear, Jackie shared an intimate detail of her arthritis.

"Do you know, some days my finger joints are so stiff that I can't

even put in and take out my tampon." She looked lovingly across at her husband. *"Then Paul does it for me."*

I was moved by this loving act of understanding and realised the high level of intimacy these two shared. Although only in their mid-20s they experienced a mature sexual joy in the midst and perhaps as a result of considerable physical limitations.

Many of my clients hope there is only a physical cause for their sexual problem, easy for the doctor to fix thus removing any need to discuss relationship and other life issues. But my clients never escape without discussion of the whole problem.

In writing this chapter, the doctor part of me struggled with concern about leaving out information on any medical condition that could interfere with sex. The therapist part wanted to put the body in context with the mind. My heart wanted to tell the stories of my clients and the human challenges that sexual problems present. Rather than describe every health problem that affects sexuality, which is a complete book in itself, I decided to give a few examples so you can get a feel for the impact of physical and mental health on sexuality. I settled on a basic diagram to explain the links. You will notice that information goes in both directions, genitals to brain, brain to genitals, etc. Everything is interwoven. And believe me this is the simplified version. You can imagine how complex the workings of the body and mind really is.

Body and mind in sex

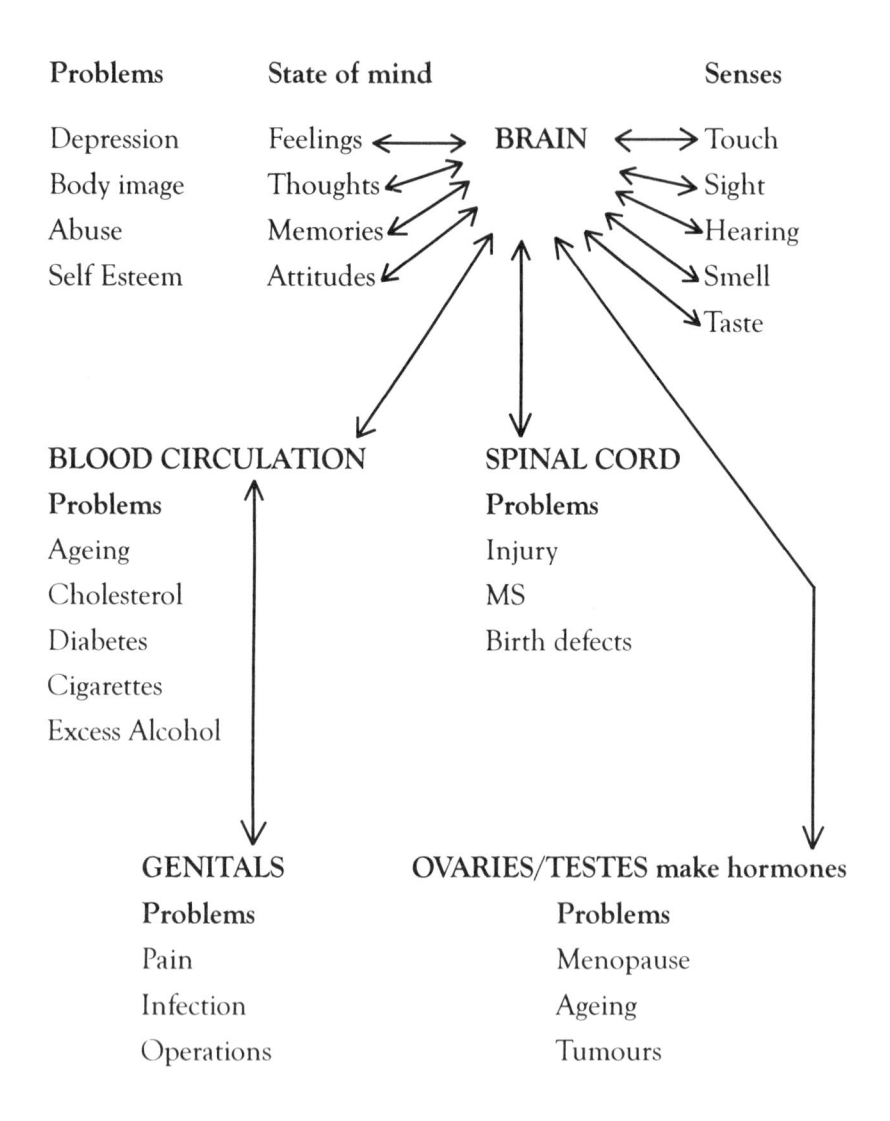

Problems	State of mind		Senses
Depression	Feelings ⟷	BRAIN ⟷	Touch
Body image	Thoughts		Sight
Abuse	Memories		Hearing
Self Esteem	Attitudes		Smell
			Taste

BLOOD CIRCULATION
Problems
Ageing
Cholesterol
Diabetes
Cigarettes
Excess Alcohol

SPINAL CORD
Problems
Injury
MS
Birth defects

GENITALS
Problems
Pain
Infection
Operations

OVARIES/TESTES make hormones
Problems
Menopause
Ageing
Tumours

Hormones

Hormones are the chemical messengers produced in glands and transmitted around the body in the blood. In women, oestrogen and progesterone vary enormously throughout each monthly cycle. Many women take the contraceptive pill, which also contains hormones. What effect do these hormones have on sexual interest? The honest truth is we do not fully understand. There are many individual variations. Some women say they feel sexier before a period, some during, some after and some not at all. The Pill can relieve anxiety about pregnancy allowing a woman to enjoy sex more. The effect may be opposite if the impact on her natural hormones sends her sex drive plummeting. Individual advice and your own perceptions are needed to find what is best for you.

Men worry about their hormones too. The production of testosterone may decrease in some men with age. But a high drive can exist with low levels of testosterone and low sex drive with high levels. It is hard to pin sexual interest to hormone levels.

Women begin to face menopause from their mid-40s. The production of hormones by the ovaries eventually ceases and a woman can be left with little oestrogen, progesterone and testosterone in her body. We do not fully understand the effect of these hormones on sexuality. Certainly some women report that they have thoroughly enjoyed sex until menopause and then found their loss of drive a problem.

However, I have found that it is not wise to assume that low hormone levels fully explain decreased interest in sex after menopause as this is not every woman's experience. In fact, some find their interest increases. On looking back clients often realised that their desire has been decreasing over a long period related to many other life factors. Menopause is a milestone but there are other 'changes of life' at the same time, children leave home, there are opportunities to return to work or study, financial change may occur and relationship problems become highlighted.

Hormone replacement therapy of oestrogen and progesterone can be terrific for overcoming symptoms of menopause – hot flushes, dry vagina, sleep disturbances and loss of bone density. Natural sources of these hormones are also being promoted. (You can find more information in the reading list).[6] But is HRT the answer to decreased interest in sex? Generally it is not.

Even more controversial is the addition of testosterone to HRT. I presented a paper to a conference in Spain in 1997[7] about the use of testosterone in women. In reviewing the research of 15 years I could see no absolute evidence that testosterone increased sexual desire (thinking and feelings of sex) in women. There was some evidence that sexual drive (basic urge) may be increased. However, a client of mine going through menopause made it very clear that testosterone treatment, given by another doctor, had not been completely beneficial for her. She told me, 'testosterone increased my interest in sex but not with my husband.'

In these few words she made it very clear where her low interest in sex lay.

Blood circulation

Touch, smell, sweet nothings in your ear, or whatever turns you on, goes straight to your brain. This sets in motion responses elsewhere in your body. Extra blood is pumped into the genitals during arousal. If circulation is good the lips of the vagina swell, the clitoris becomes hard and the penis becomes erect.

However, many men experience erection problems at different times in life. By the age of 60 up to 50% of men have had a period of erectile difficulty though this has often been temporary. We know plenty about blood flow in erections because it is obvious to a man himself if everything is working or not. In addition, machines can measure blood flow in and out of the penis. For a woman there is less to see and very little research into female arousal to promote further understanding. As a result the range of treatments available are focused on problems in men. Injections, pumps and pills are available, though they can improve the physical response there is no guarantee they alter sexual satisfaction which involves much more than simply getting stiff.

Patricia and Bill show how complex are the factors, which impact on arousal. They came to see me some months after Bill had a heart attack. He was 64.

"I'm too worried to have sex with Bill. What if he has another heart attack in the middle? I'd never forgive myself," explained Pat.

"What a way to go." Bill tried to make light of her concern.

"I couldn't bear to have him grab his chest in pain or stop breathing while we were making love. It's too horrible." Patricia let the grief she had been holding in for months out in a torrent of howls.

"There now, Pet. I know how you feel, I've been worried too." Bill patted her knee. He looked awkwardly at me for help.

I asked him if he had any other concerns about his recovery. I wondered even if he had would he voice them?

"No, the specialist says I'm going well. The coronary artery by-pass has been great. I've had no chest pain since."

I explained that if the arteries to his heart had become clogged then arteries elsewhere in his body might also be affected, including the ones into his penis. Had he noticed any change in his erections?

"I don't get hard like I used to. In fact, I don't often get an erection even when I wake up. I was beginning to wonder what was happening."

Bill had begun to talk about what worries many men. Pat had

thought her concern about the effect of sex on his heart was the cause of the problem.

"I thought you weren't getting erections because I told you I didn't think sex was a good idea at the moment. You never said you had noticed a change in your self."

Pat was surprised that he had not told her that his concern was not his heart but his penis.

"Well, I hoped it would get better," Bill muttered.

"You are a silly thing," said Pat. *"I love you to bits. I'm happy that you're alive and fairly well. I would like to have sex with you. I can think of lots of things that we could do without an erection."*

"Now you surprise me," Bill joked.

Pat was reassured that as Bill was walking up and down the stairs several times a day without any chest pain his heart was already handling more physical effort than he would expend during sex. He had certainly had a warning about his health but nothing that should limit his pleasure in living. But Pat needed to talk through her fears for the future and have them acknowledged by Bill. It also helped Bill to recognise his own concerns.

Talking about their fears of loss brought them closer as they came in touch with the depth of the love that they felt for each other. They realised they had a choice to make. They could live in fear of Bill's heart condition or they could rejoice in having each other in the present. They chose to enjoy their here and now but did choose to reduce any undue exertion.

They had always used the missionary position with Bill on top. They now found that they were both less worried if he lay back in a comfortable position supported by pillows and their lovemaking was gentle with Pat putting in more of the physical effort. She found this exciting and had plenty of ideas that she had never been game to try before. They found a renewed eroticism at this late stage in life with their new sexual style and developed a full sexual life. Bill's erections actually improved as he relaxed and enjoyed himself. They decided not to worry about what might be.

Eventually Bill did die. He was aged 73 and sitting in a chair. Pat talked to me after Bill's death about their 9 years of sexual joy.

"Do you know we discovered all kinds of positions and played around in ways we'd never have dreamed of before Bill's heart attack? It was as though we realised that it was now or never. We decided to do whatever took our fancy. It was fun. I wouldn't have missed it for the world."

This philosophy surely holds true whatever your age and whatever your state of health.

Nerve connections

During sex, blood is directed to rush into the genitals by impulses from the brain, carried in the nerves. Injury or disease of the nervous system can disturb this flow and cause a problem with sexual responses.

Craig, aged 28, had been an active sportsman when he was struck down with an infection in his brain. For some time afterwards Craig was paralysed down one side of his body. With much effort on his part and support from his wife, Maggie, he regained good movement. However, since the illness he had ceased to have erections at any time.

"Life has been difficult. I've had to deal with losing my job, my energy, most of our hopes and dreams. But I've been able to find other things to do. We bought a small house with two acres of land and we grow enough food to be self-sufficient. I like that we spend more time together. It was difficult at first but I am enjoying being with Maggie and doing heaps with our 3-year-old, Toby."

Craig and Maggie talked extensively about the significant adaptations they had made. It was clear they had a strong relationship.

Their mutual love and respect had deepened as a result of this considerable challenge.

"We came to see you to find out if there was any way that Craig could have erections again. We're OK with sex but he gets fed up sometimes because even when he's turned on his penis stays soft.

"I haven't had an erection since the brain damage. Maggie says she doesn't mind but there was something very special about being inside her. It was like a special union between us. I miss that." He sighed. *Maggie leaned over to reach for the tissues.*

This is when I appreciate my medical training. I thought it possible that medication could provide what they wanted. After all their difficulties it was a delight to discuss with them the various options available. A chemical message normally passes from the brain through the nervous system to the penis in response to stimulation. Craig's brain was no longer able to do this. A drug, Sildenafil, can be taken which bypasses the brain and acts directly on the penis. There was hope of a good response. Craig took a prescription and tried the tablets at home. Both he and Maggie were over the moon with the response.

I saw them occasionally over the next few months to monitor treatment.

"At first I was like a kid in a sweet shop. But as I settled down, there were times we wanted to share intercourse and times we wanted the kind of sex we'd had before the tablets. It's great to have the choice."

Craig's smile was reward indeed. Maggie squeezed Craig's hand, "We take what each day brings. Some days that's a lot."

Medicine has a valuable role to play when practiced in the context of the whole person. There are many health problems that impact on sexuality in both a physical and emotional ways.

If you are experiencing any sexual difficulties and think that your physical health may be involved, then do seek medical advice.

State of mind

Since body and mind are interconnected it is obvious that your state of mind is a major influence on sexual function. Whenever your mind is not at peace, for whatever reason, neither is your body. The more severe illnesses of the mind have a clear effect on the body.

Depression

Unfortunately, clinical depression is a common diagnosis and disinterest in many activities, including sex, frequently accompanies depression. Feeling good is important for feeling sexy; in contrast, depression has the same impact as an icy cold dip.

Post Natal Depression (PND) may be associated with hormonal change and can contribute to a decline in sexual drive. But there are other factors impacting on mental health at this tumultuous time. The responsibilities of caring for a dependent baby and disturbed nights have their own dampening effect on both parents, even in the absence of depression. But should sexual problems persist longer than these disruptions, it is timely to seek help.

Treatments for depression can in themselves cause sexual problems for instance some newer anti-depressants (the SSRI's) can cause delayed ejaculation. There are reports of a multitude of other medications interfering with sexual responses. Again, if you feel that any medication you are taking is affecting your sexual responses do talk to your doctor.

Anxiety

Anxiety is an ancient response of the body to danger. You remain alert and ready to fight or flee as though under attack. This was a lifesaver when the danger was a huge animal about to devour you for his supper. Now anxiety is more likely to result from worry caused by less threatening problems.

It may come as a shock to many men to know that their psyche is involved in erection. The experience of teenage years of erections being automatic leaves a strong memory. Many young men do not need direct touch on the penis to get an erection. It can happen with embarrassing ease, simply by eyeing a girl at the beach. Perhaps this results from a combination of high circulating testosterone in the years around puberty and joy in anticipation of sex without the complications of long-term relationship and a more serious lifestyle.

Yet some young men will have erection difficulties usually related to pressure to perform. Unfortunate circumstances within a relationship, concerns about the size of the penis or how long an erection will last - all of these performance factors can cause anxiety. The problem with too much anxiety is that the brain assumes you are in danger. Adrenaline is released which diverts blood into areas of the body, essential for fleeing from danger, particularly the leg muscles. Your brain thinks that an erection is useless in saving your life and so reduces blood flow to the penis.

Then to add to erectile problems, starting around age 40 more genital touch is generally required to obtain an erection, probably due to reduced reaction in the nerve fibres and blood vessels to stimulation. Many men do not realise this is normal and may worry that their penises are not responding as they did years before. This can create a vicious cycle of anxiety and even less erectile response.

If you think that this is all about men's sexuality, unfortunately you are correct. This stems from the physical obviousness of a sex problem in men. If a man cannot get an erection, he cannot have sexual intercourse. Women, however, can easily hide any lack of arousal by using a lubricating gel and even faking orgasm as the famous scene in the movie, 'When Harry Meets Sally', demonstrated. This fraud, often well intentioned to protect a partner from feeling hurt, means arousal difficulties in women can go unnoticed. If you do this, you cheat your self out of the opportunity to be honest with your partner and to enjoy better sex. Perhaps as a result less is known about the physical impact of anxiety on sexual responses in women. Being honest would not only improve scientific knowledge but also the truth factors in a sexual relationship.

Sexual worries may stem from physical problems including surgery to treat breast cancer, hysterectomy, prostate surgery and many other operations and illnesses as well as a multitude of mental concerns. Being anxious is the opposite of being relaxed. Yet relaxation is an essential part of sexual sharing in couples. Whatever the reason for the anxiety (even when you do not know the cause your self) help is worth considering. Many of these anxieties can be relieved by talking to someone who you think will understand, a therapist, doctor, support group or friend.

Sexual abuse

Sexual abuse in the past can contribute to anxiety about sex. Feelings, smells, or the touch of sex in the present can trigger unpleasant memories of abuse in the past. These triggers can be very specific, such as a touch on the breast that links the present with the past. Your reaction can send you reeling backwards. Not only are you upset but it can be difficult for your partner to understand your response to sex with him/her, knowing he/she is not the abuser. These complex difficulties require some help.[8]

Body image

This particular cause of anxiety has enormous sway on your sexuality. Do you look in the mirror to decide if you are attractive or not? Are you (or have you been) concerned about the size and shape of your body? Inevitably you are responding to a culture that reveres the tall, slender, beautiful, young person. These attributes are linked with sexiness and promoted by a multi-million dollar advertising industry.

Kaz Cooke, author of the book, *Real Gorgeous*, made this comment on a recent ABC radio interview about the philosophy of sales. "If we all had thin thighs they'd be promoting cream to make our thighs fat." It makes economic sense to be selling a product that promises to change you from the way you are into something you are not. You have to buy an awful lot of the stuff! Yet women buy anti-wrinkle cream and cellulite reduction pills, spend millions on dieting substances and cosmetic surgery. Whatever happened to celebrating the assets of the body you have.

Many women are extremely miserable about their body size. Geneen Roth in her book, *Appetites*,[9] reported:

> *In a recent survey in 'Esquire magazine', a thousand women were asked whether they would rather be run over by a truck or gain one hundred and fifty pounds. 54.3% answered that they would rather be run over by a truck... Because the size of their bodies determines the quality of their lives, they would rather be dead than fat.*

The Body Shop recently printed T-shirts that stated, 'There are 3 billion women who don't look like supermodels and only 8 who do'. Yet many are hooked into the theory that being thin and young equates to being sexy.

Many years ago when I worked in a women's health clinic I had clients who appeared on television or were models. Their common lifestyle was to workout in the gym several hours a day, eat lettuce at meals, and have terrible love relationships. They were rarely comfortable with themselves, they were not satisfied with their bodies nor did they know sexual self-esteem. Yet they were role models for young people. I have never known someone to go to extremes to be thin, purely for the cosmetic appearance and be happy for a prolonged period of time.

Young men today are falling into the same trap and spend more time worrying about their body shape and the size of body parts. Plastic surgery is thriving to plump out shoulders and even extend the length of penises. Steroid use to build muscles is not only a temptation for Olympic athletes but also for guys at the local gym.

Did you look in the mirror today and say, "You're looking good," or did you stand there focused on a roll of fat, a dimple of cellulite and hate your self? If you did the latter, it is difficult to celebrate your physical body in sex. Conformity to a fixed body shape does not allow you to be your self. Slender or voluptuous, feeling good about your whole self is essential for being desirous and desirable sexually.

Part of your truth is your genetic inheritance – blue eyes, red hair, big nose, short, rounded, whatever characteristics are the real you. If you are trying to alter your body deliberately with starvation, vomiting or overeating, use of drugs or abuse of alcohol you exude a desperation to be someone else. On the other hand when you are at ease within your self you radiate an attraction that is as magnetic as nectar to a bee. Your body is part of the total package of body, mind and spirit, programmed from your conception. Fight your self and you cannot be happy. Find your self, accept all of your self and you can be.

As you read further in this book about people facing the challenges of love and sex, you will see how little the externals of body size and age have to do with their happiness.

If you have any concerns about sexual function, ask a doctor you feel comfortable with to check your health. Book a long appointment as this takes time. Several books[10] provide more detail of health problems that can affect sex than is possible to include here.

If you decide to seek a therapist your choice of therapist is very important. You want someone who will respect your individuality and help you work through the problems in a way that makes sense to you. There are organisations you can contact for further details.[11]

Only flesh and blood?

*I have dreamed a wonderful dream; of life and love...
A wonderful dream, my many – splendoured thing.*

'A Many Splendoured Thing'
Han Suyin

Chapter Six

What is this thing called love?

This may seem like a silly question. You know what love is but do other people have the same concept of love that you do? If you are planning to embark on the voyage called love and sex you need to be clear about both these subjects. There are many different types of love yet there is only one word 'love' to describe an amazing variety of experiences. When I was young and was not sure of the meaning of a word, I was told to look it up in a dictionary. Using this wisdom, I found three distinct definitions of 'love'.

1. A feeling of great affection and devotion to another person. The affection that exists between lover and sweetheart and is the normal basis of marriage.

2. A strong sexual passion for another person. The personification of sexual affection, the animal instinct between the sexes and its gratification.

This definition of love might surprise you. You may call this lust. But the *Oxford Dictionary (Compact)* has no such qualms. Gratification of sexual drive is a definition of love.

3. A feeling of warm personal attachment or deep affection, as for a friend or family member. A feeling with regard to a person (arising from recognition of attractive qualities from instincts of natural relationship or from sympathy) which manifests itself in the solicitude for the welfare of the object and usually the delight in his or her presence and desire for his or her approval.

It is interesting to see here the thinking of the compiler of the dictionary. For he reflects the view of many that love involves the desire for approval by someone else rather than self-approval.

The English language has one word for love but three distinct meanings. The ancient Greeks made their lives easier by using three different words for love:

1. *Agape* – heart to heart love.
2. *Eros* – sexual love.
3. *Philia* – friendship or fraternal love.

Using these Greek concepts you can develop some clear guidelines for understanding the life-changing words, 'I love you'. They could mean:

1. I feel *Agape* for you. – 'I feel deep affection for you.'
2. I feel *Eros* for you. – 'I fancy you sexually.'
3. I feel *Philia* for you. – 'I feel an attachment and care about your welfare.'

If you recall Justin and Leanne (page 20), they both said 'I love you'. But Justin felt 'Eros' and Leanne felt 'Agape'. They could have saved themselves a lot of pain if both had been clear about their different emotions before deciding to have sex together.

Have you ever misunderstood a declaration of 'love'? Have you had sex only to be disappointed later that their love was not the same as your love? You can avoid this particular heartache if you make sure you know what sort of love you are each feeling.

I have found it useful to compose some other definitions for distinct types of love. You can use these to recognise exactly how you feel for someone and how they feel for you. The exercise at the end of this chapter will help you to compare the types of love you have for those close to you.

Unconditional love

Unconditional love requires the ability to recognise the beauty within another, but also acknowledge their behaviour may not be as lovely. If you were able to see the good within and ignore everything else then it would be possible to love everyone. It is the way that people like Mother Theresa love. For those less saintly you may be unable to see beneath disrespectful behaviour. But even unconditional love does not excuse bad behaviour. Each person must take full responsibility for how they act.

You meet thousands of people during life, yet experience love for only a few. What makes the difference? In addition to unconditional love you have preferences for the behaviour and thinking that you like. You can love someone but not like his or her behaviour.

You might find your self in a real dilemma for instance if you 'fall in love' with someone who has a kind personality but later turns out to be violent when drunk. Ken Keyes'[12] definition of unconditional love is helpful in understanding the confusion of feelings that can result:

Unconditional love is the ability to separate the person from their behaviour. The only way one can love unconditionally is to distinguish between a person and their programming which causes the person's behaviour.

It takes unconditional love **and** liking to maintain a long-term relationship.

You may find it easier to be able to make this separation between the essential beauty of the inner person and their behaviour if you keep in mind that there are different types of love.

Dependent love

The first love you experience is the love of your parents for their helpless infant. Love begins with a 100% dependency on your parents to provide the essentials of life, not only food and shelter but also tender touch.

As an infant you expect unlimited access to love and unlimited giving by your carer. Of course this childhood dream is impossible for parents to totally fulfil. The less love is available the more you, as a child, become aware of a scarcity of love. You learn how to get more of what you want, be it with a smile, a gurgle, or something else of which your parent approves. You develop your ways to get as much love as possible.

In teenage years and early adulthood when you want to be loved by another you subconsciously tap into early lessons on love, triggered by your own questions – What must I do to get love, to get approval, to get my needs met?

Dependent love originates from a continuation of your childhood desire to hold onto and own the supply of love because you remember that love is scarce.

Dependent love thus is possessive (he/she is mine) as you try to hold on to the only supply you know – someone else. If you expect all the love you need to come from someone else, there can never be enough.

As each year passes dependency on your parents should reduce. Ideally by the time you are an adult and ready to leave home you have obtained full independence. In the practical areas of providing your own food and shelter this may be so, for these you received useful lessons on taking care of your self. But what lessons did you receive on being able to love your self?

Early lessons, limited by the experience of your various teachers rarely go this far. You can be an adult yet be inadequately prepared to reach your full potential for loving and the sexual expression of love. You might get stuck for years at the stage of dependent love.

> *You need me*
> *And I need you*
> *Without each other*
> *There ain't nothing you can do.*
>
> 'Think'
> Aretha Franklin & Ted White

You have to take the next steps for your self along the path to mature love.

It can be difficult to view your thoughts and feelings about love as a maturing process. But it is incompleteness in this passage that has much to do with the frequent dissatisfaction in love and sex.

Provisional love

Provisional love is the love limited by how little two people know of each other. When you are unsure of your self and are unwilling to reveal your all, you are limited to provisional love. You may feel the powerful mixture of Agape and Eros. This may be the foundation of a long-term affiliation. But you will be restricted to Provisional Love until you are ready to bare your selves to each other. Only then can love develop the open honesty of knowing and being known.

Mature love

Mature love is the love and respect of your self, which you can choose to share with another. It grows from loving and liking someone. You have fully opened your hearts and minds to each other. You have striven to respect your differences. Each has taken responsibility for recognising their limiting patterns of behaviour. Each has been willing to change and grow. Each has decided what they wish to change for their own benefit. The relationship allows the two to grow faster than either would alone.

> *Love has an infinite heart*
> *and cannot grow in a narrow mind.*
> *It is always sweeping on and on*
> *always living, growing and becoming.*
> *And those who have stopped*
> *changing and growing*
> *have stopped loving.*
>
> 'Celebrating Love'
> Mary Hathaway, 1993

This growth is important for the full enjoyment of Philia, Agape or Eros. In mature Philia (friendship or fraternal love) you come to lovingly acknowledge the limitations of family members. You understand what and why they were able and also unable to provide. Independent of parents you can obtain for your self, from within and through your own endeavours, what you still desire. In doing so you can experience love for your parents even if you do not like all their behaviour. From love, not resentment, anger or need, you decide the nature of the time you wish to spend with them.

Mature Agape and Eros are joyous when both can celebrate who they really are in each other's presence. Maturity in love and sexuality can accommodate changes in life, in the body with ageing, in the world in which you live and changes in the connection and desires of each other.

A mature adult expects no one else to provide for them. Mature love is not love given and received but love shared. Thus, mature love cannot be possessed. It cannot be given or taken away. It exists in the present. Mature love is the love based on personal freedom.

> *If I have freedom in my love*
> *and in my soul am free,*
> *angels alone that soar above*
> *enjoy such liberty.*
>
> Richard Lovelace, 1618-1658

Dysfunctional love

Dysfunctional love is based on a failure to be able to separate love from need. Love and need are not the same. Yet needs being met by another can easily be mistaken for love. When you love someone you respect them and appreciate they will change over time.

> *If we keep someone from growth we must immediately examine our 'love'.*
>
> 'Born to Love'
> Leo Buscaglia, 1992

If you take what you need in disregard of another, the love is dysfunctional because there is a lack of equality and respect. A person holding power can appear to love someone in a less powerful position and use their position for their own advantage.

This misuse of power results in the abuse of the powerless but this is a game of power not love. It may be deliberate and occur at a conscious level.

> *I love you. You are so beautiful and intelligent. I can make sure you get promotion. I want to have sex with you.*
>
> Company executive to employee

More commonly, dysfunctional love begins at a more subtle unconscious level. Both are unaware of the relevance of one having more knowledge, money, position or authority than the other, yet this power is used for sexual advantage. Ignorance of a power differential is not an acceptable reason to gain from it and some professions make sure their members are aware. It is unethical for a doctor to become sexually involved with a patient. It is wrong for a therapist to fall in love with a client. You need the same awareness for your self even in less obvious circumstances.

Are there any circumstances in which you or your partner misuse your power to gain what you want at the expense of the other?

> "*I'll take you out for an expensive dinner (which I know you can't afford but I can) if you...*"

There is always an implicit condition attached to the seemingly innocent offer. Sex is a common playground of these unhappy games.

> *"I'll find someone else (which I know you don't want) unless you give me sex."*
>
> *"I'd just love a holiday in the sun let me show you how much..."*

A relationship rooted in inequality will eventually change when the person lower on the power scale begins to feel uncomfortable and seek equality. Commonly this results in conflict. The power broker will try to maintain their position and may resort to some style of emotional blackmail.

This power game of dysfunctional love also exists in some families.

Parents may enforce their own desires in the name of love on their children.

> *No one will ever love you like I love you, David.*
>
> Father of the pianist, David Helfgott, on refusing to let his talented son attend the Academy of Music.
> 'Shine' 1996 (Movie)

A child can also manipulate a parent into sacrificing his or her own wants to gain the child's love.

> *"All the other parents have bought their kids one of these (which I know you can't afford). If you loved me you would too."*

Any adult who acts on their sexual feelings toward a child and calls this love is at the extreme of dysfunction. In fact, they are completely abusing the child's trust for an adult. The perpetrator can be unaware of the reality of the power differential that exists and still use words of love.

> *I love that boy so much I will do anything legal to see him again – even if I only see him through the day and bring him back at night.*
>
> Extract from letter sent by a jailed paedophile
to the mother of the boy he abused
Courier Mail, Brisbane, 1997

This use of the word love is particularly common in the tragedy of incest. It is vital to make some distinctions about different types of love or that one word can cloak abusive behaviour.

Making love

You may use the term 'making love' to describe sexual intercourse. Couples often say, "We don't have sex (Eros), we make love (Agape and Eros)," to show they feel both a physical and emotional bond during intercourse. But have you ever done things the other way round and had sex to make love? You found your self attracted to someone and were needy of love so you had sex.

Justin and Leanne (page 20) were a good example of this:

Eros:	"Do you want to have sex?" exhaled Justin.
Agape:	"Do you love me?" inhaled Leanne.
Eros:	"Oh Yes," Justin panted. "I love you."
Agape & Eros:	Leanne melted into making love.

Leanne was making love. Could this be the origin of this phrase? Do you want sex with a loved one to be a 'making' or occur as a desired erotic connection? Words can be funny things.

Divine love

There is one love that is not about the love between two people. It is the love inside your self. It is your Self, the very core of you. Divine love can nourish your life. But unfortunately it is a most neglected love, the one you may rarely rely upon. Your own spiritual belief will decide what you call this - Joy, Essence, Self Trust, Self Esteem, Divine, God (Buddha, Allah, Jehovah, etc.), Spirit, Soul or Universal Awareness. This is the love you may overlook as you rush headlong in your search for love received from another. You may even suspect that self love is indulgently narcistic. Uncomfortable with feeling good about your self from the inside you instead seek love from others. However, at some point in life - often as a result of crisis - you turn inwards to utilise your inner strength. Unconditional love and mature love flow from this core.

I began to trust in love once
I slowly came to know, that my deeper soul
is pulsed by an eternal flow.

The Eternal Heartbeat
Stuart Wilde

What do you mean by love?

What are you experiencing when you love someone? This question opens up much for you to consider, when you thought you already knew what love was. You can appreciate there are many ways to love. With these definitions you can become clearer about what love means to you.

You will find your ideas fall into place as you complete the following two tables. The first table is your assessment of the type of love you have for each person that you name. The second is your view of how you think they love you.

You can tick as many boxes as you like against each name you have entered. Later as you ponder on this you may want to write your own individual definition of the love you want to experience.

How do I love you?

	First name	Agape	Eros	Philia	Unconditional	Provisional	Mature	Dependent	Dysfunctional
Spouse/-partner									
Children									
Mum									
Dad									
Sisters									
Brothers									
Friends									
Others									

WHAT IS THIS THING CALLED LOVE?

How do you love me?

First name	Agape	Eros	Philia	Unconditional	Provisional	Mature	Dependent	Dysfunctional
Spouse/-partner								
Children								
Mum								
Dad								
Sisters								
Brothers								
Friends								
Others								

Part Two

Embarking on the Love Boat

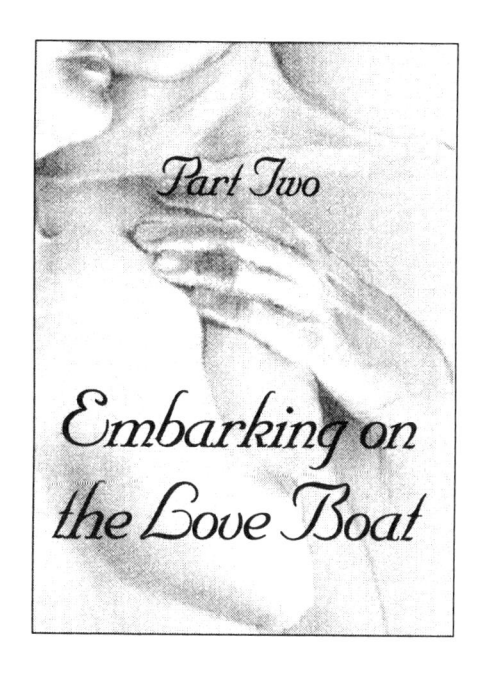

The Owl and the Pussy-Cat went to sea
In a beautiful pea-green boat,
They took some honey and plenty of money,
Wrapped up in a five pound note.

They sailed away for a year and a day...

The Owl and the Pussy-Cat
Edward Lear

Lovers at first sight
In love forever.
It turned out so right
For strangers in the night.

'Strangers in the Night'
Bert Kaemfert, Charles Singleton, Eddie Snyder

Chapter Seven

The honeymoon suite

You embark on the love boat fuelled with passion, ready to check into the honeymoon suite for the cruise of a lifetime. You booked your passage to celebrate falling 'in love', the common beginning of many voyages of love and sex. Our culture is hooked on 'falling in love'. We adore 'they lived happily ever after' endings. Fairy tales such as Cinderella capture our hearts. Movies like 'Pretty Woman' (with the unlikely story of a sophisticated, wealthy man who falls in love with a beautiful prostitute) are often smash hits. Romantic novels are also very popular worldwide. In Australia Mills and Boon are the most purchased and read books. Poems and songs about being in love have been popular for centuries. Yet what happens next is largely ignored.

No one has dared to make a realistic movie sequel to a romantic love story. I wonder how 'Pretty Woman II' (five years later on) would really be. Would he be complaining of her lack of manners and would she be telling him he is a workaholic?

Does part of you cling to the hope that 'happily ever after' will be yours? Is this embedded in your unconscious even though you know, in real life, there are a lot of unhappy relationships and unhappy sex?

If you choose 'in love' to be the first stage of a long-term relationship. You will need to give some thought to the possible sequels as well as the heart-felt delights. You may have known the sexual excitement of being 'in love'. It is wonderful to enjoy a sexual romance but you also need to remember that this is only the first stage of love relationships. There is more to come!

Falling in love is a time of delightful and powerful emotions. But do you enter commitment prematurely? Are you desperate to hang on to the happiness of being 'in love'? Marianne and Joe were.

Marianne and Joe started their relationship 'in love'. They came to see me during their first holiday together, on the Sunshine Coast in Australia, where I live. Joe was 29, Marianne was 25. They had both had a couple of long term relationships before meeting each other 10 months previous. It was unusual to have a couple request to see me so early in a relationship but they had a problem. I asked them to begin by talking about their early days together.

Poised on the edge of her seat, Marianne began.

"When I first met Joe I hadn't hoped for too much. I wondered if the few glasses of wine at the party had encouraged him to show some interest. But Joe 'phoned me. Our first date was fun. I spent a long time choosing what to wear. I remember taking time arranging my hair. Should I put it up or leave it down? Did I want to look sophisticated or casual? I chose down. It was the right choice. I just knew it, when I opened the door that night. Joe looked cool and casual in a clean linen shirt, though I remembered he had looked a bit scruffy at the party."

Joe broke into a smile as he also remembered that night. "I was out to impress you," he said.

"The first three weeks of dates were terrific. I looked forward to finishing work. I'd rush home and get ready. All I wanted to do was to

be with Joe. I loved spending time getting ready. I hadn't felt that way for a long time. It was worth it because Joe noticed the way I dressed. I remember the smell of his after shave. It was a knockout."

I could sense the delight they had felt. But I could also appreciate the context of their dating that had contributed to everything being so enjoyable. Joe and Marianne had their own lives when they met. They lived separately, in their own apartments. Each time they met was special. There was preparation for the date, showering, special clothes, and special plans to do something together. The joy of the effort to create pleasurable situations in fact seemed effortless. Trips, movies, dinners, picnics, walks, sharing sunsets all added to the enchantment of being 'in love'. It was so intoxicating that Marianne and Joe stopped seeing other friends and spent leisure time only with each other.

Marianne continued:

"We had a weekend free, Joe suggested we go to the beach. As we drove towards the beach I thought of the day ahead. Lunch on the beach a swim and 'who knows what else?'

"Usually I avoided the beach. I need to be careful with my fair skin not to burn. Joe loved surfing and was tanned so brown. I packed sunscreen oil and a hat and hoped I'd be OK. I didn't want Joe to think I was silly, fussing about my skin."

Joe was dying to join in with his own memory.

"I was also thinking of lunch on the beach a swim and who knows what else? Marianne had prepared the picnic. I hoped she hadn't made Thai salad. I wasn't keen on the hot chillies she liked. She said she'd spent ages preparing the food so I didn't want to say anything. I really didn't care. It wasn't important. Everything else was going so well."

I saw what they could not at the time, when they were pulsing with enthusiasm for the relationship. 'In love' Joe and Marianne made every effort to please each other. For themselves neither would have chosen what the other wanted. But for the enjoyment of love it did not seem worthwhile to disagree and voice their preferences. The approval of the other was of utmost importance. Each unconsciously willed themselves to be what the other desired.

"*I felt like I had known Joe forever. I felt warm, wrapped in his arms. I felt safe to share my thoughts. It was so wonderful to find someone I could share everything with. We had so much in common. We were made for each other. I remember saying to Joe that I couldn't think of a single difference between us. Joe had laughed and said, 'I know something. I just love surfing and I know you don't.'*

"*I told him he was mistaken. When I was a child I always wanted a surfboard for Christmas. My parents wouldn't let me have one. They said surfing was too dangerous.*"

"*I offered to teach her.*" Joe beamed proudly.

I could imagine them on the beach, day dreaming the bliss of their sameness. 'In love' both were overwhelmed by their visible similarities. Marianne and Joe clearly enjoyed being together. It appeared a delight for both to eat Thai food, for both to surf. But Joe did not like Thai food and Marianne did not enjoy going to the beach – before they met. Their relationship developed based on the many interests they apparently shared.

Marianne sped on:

"*Since meeting that first time at the party we knew it would lead to sex. As we had both been hurt before we had decided not to rush. But each date was getting more 'heavy'. It was hard to wait three weeks. Then it seemed like a lifetime.*

"*But that day at the beach was just right. Joe was so thoughtful. He drove across the city to pick me up. He took me to his special hideaway. He had bought some chilled wine and I had prepared a feast. The view across the secluded beach was magic. We played around in the water and one thing led to another. You know what I mean."*

I did know, I had seen the movie. Joe and Marianne were in Eros. Their delight touched my own memories of this exciting time but also the memories of the many possible routes that 'in love' can take.

At the stage of 'in love' relationships are often full of expectancy for sexual satisfaction in the flush of early attraction. Sexual interest is often high as a result of the joy of finding a person who seems to match you. Sex may be frequent and enjoyable with heightened sensations.

Attraction can be an opening guide to the potential for a relationship. But it is not always easy to remember to separate the lusty effects of sexual drive from long-term compatibility. The possibility for full intimacy can rarely be gauged from these first few meetings. The initial sexual attraction, the falling in lust, may be a vital part of the reproduction of the species but it is insufficient for long-term pleasure. It needs to be accompanied by much more.

Added to the sexual attraction is the attraction of finding someone new. Anything new that you choose, be it a car, a house, a dress or a lover has novelty. This adds to the experience of 'in love'.

Marianne and Joe had been in a hurry. With the ingredients they found it would have been hard for Marianne and Joe not to fall in love. They illustrate the essentials of being 'in love':

- pleasing each other
- making an effort in getting ready for a date, special places, etc
- sexual attraction
- apparent sameness
- novelty
- isolation from friends

A couple 'in love' become residents of the honeymoon suite. This is a haven where there is only awareness of their love. It is a beautiful place separated from the outside world by an enveloping mist. Love in the mist allows only a fuzzy view of each other. Wedding albums (my own included) often contain photos taken through a lens that softens the definition of the faces. The couple looks gorgeous but the picture is a blurring of the truth.

You may be wondering why Joe and Marianne had come to see me. Unlike the Hollywood version of 'in love' which automatically guarantees great sex, Joe and Marianne had experienced a problem with sex from the beginning.

"I 'came' very quickly that day," Joe squirmed. *"I know Marianne was disappointed. We said nothing. I hoped it was because it was our first time for intercourse with each other. But it hasn't got any better. I didn't know what to say or do. It's never been a problem for me before."*

"I couldn't say anything. I didn't want to hurt his feelings," Marianne admitted.

I had heard this comment many times before and each time it had resulted in more anxiety rather than less. This fear of hurting Joe contributed to the problem not being dealt with. Joe did not understand why he was 'coming' (ejaculating) so fast with Marianne. He did not want to but then he did not want to talk about it either. 'In love' preferences and concerns are often not stated for fear they may hurt the other person. What we really fear is that we may lose the relationship with the other person if we reveal what we would really like. This fear interferes with the growth of integrity and honesty in a relationship. It is essential to overcome this fear and to be able to say what you think and feel to the person with whom you are relating. The sooner this fear is tackled the easier the outcome.

The skill required is the same whether you are telling a friend what you think of her new dress or talking to your lover during sex. It does take practice to be able to say what you like or prefer and feel comfortable. If you are being honest with a kind heart, allow the response of the other person to be their responsibility. If the other feels 'hurt' then that is an issue for them to address.

Consider how you feel as you read each response in the examples on the next two pages. Which style of response is the one you would like to make? Warm-hearted dishonesty often feels the easiest. It is the path that Marianne and Joe followed. As a result their problems remained unresolved.

If your intent is to be honest and true to your self but are unsure how to do this – you could try the 'Honesty With Tact' approach outlined in the following table:

Saying what you feel with honesty and tact
Responses from a cold heart

General

Jane asks, *"Do you like my new dress?"*
Her friend could reply:

| **Brutally honest** | **Judgmental** | **Put down** |
| No! | No. It doesn't suit you. | No. You look terrible. |

Mother asks, *"Do you like the jumper I've knitted for you?"*
Her son could reply:

| **Brutally honest** | **Judgmental** | **Put down** |
| No! | No. It's the wrong pattern. | No. You're a hope less knitter. Why do you waste your time? |

During sex

Marianne asks, *"Do you like me doing this?"*
Joe could reply:

| **Brutally honest** | **Judgmental** | **Put down** |
| No! | No. You don't know a thing. | No. Jenny knew exactly what to do to please me. |

Joe asks, *"Did I 'come' too quickly?"*
Marianne could reply:

| **Brutally honest** | **Judgmental** | **Put down** |
| Yes! | Yes. You're a jerk. | Yes you did. Philip could last for ages. |

Responses from a warm heart

Dishonest	**Honesty and tact**	**Stating your preference**
Yes, it's lovely.	It's a lovely colour.	I prefer to see you in a more floaty/fitted dress.
Dishonest	**Honesty and tact**	**Stating your preference**
Yes it's lovely.	Thank you, I appreciate the time you took.	I would like you to knit me another jumper. Here's the pattern and colour wool that I would really like.

Dishonest	**Honesty and tact**	**Stating your preference**
Yes it's lovely.	I prefer it if you touched me here – like this.	I like different touch at different times. I'd like to tell you what I like - at the time. I'd like to know what you like too.
Dishonest	**Honesty and tact**	**Stating your preference**
No. It was lovely.	I liked what you were doing before you came but I haven't come yet – let's do some more.	I'd like to try it more slowly next time. Would that be difficult for you? I know it takes a while to get used to each other.

Later in the consultation Marianne leaned forward with her arms tightly crossed:

"Joe has been stressed out at work. I hoped a relaxing time on holiday would sort things out. Joe spent most of his time surfing and hardly anytime with me."

"You could have come surfing," Joe spat back.

"You know I get sunburnt," Marianne pouted.

I asked them to continue with why they had come to see me when they were on holiday.

"We had a terrible argument about sex. Joe stormed out of the apartment. When he got back we hardly spoke to each other. I was scared by the argument. I told Faye, a girlfriend of mine who lives here. She suggested we see you."

"We thought you might have a cure for the problem," Joe enthusiastically added.

I felt Joe's desperate plea for a quick fix. But their problem was not only about premature ejaculation (coming too fast). I thought this was likely to be the symptom, not the cause of the problem.

The underlying cause was the anxiety Joe felt about the relationship. He was spurred on by sexual interest and his emotions but the relationship was moving faster than he was ready for – at a thinking level.

Anxiety is a problem that affects the mind and the body. It is often expressed as a sexual problem.

It became clear that Marianne and Joe knew little of what lay inside each other's minds. They had concerns but were unable to talk about and share them.

Although they had been together for 10 months, the significance of their differences had only just begun to dawn on them. But they had already made a commitment.

"I moved out from my apartment and changed my job to live with you," said Marianne.

" I know." Joe hung his head.

The anxiety associated with the premature commitment meant the premature ejaculation persisted. They had a lot of thinking to do.

When I counsel a couple like Marianne and Joe, disillusioned after being 'in love', I am always saddened by their disappointment. I have a sincere hope that you will come to appreciate that 'in love' is a lovely time but holds no assurances of compatibility. Perhaps Hollywood might make some movies that fill us with the joy of real love stories. The ones that take time to mature – not the fantasy of forever being born in the twinkling of a starlit night.

This is not to deny the joy of romantic love. Time in the honeymoon suite is exciting and special but it involves high emotion and low levels of thinking. If you are planning long-term commitment it pays to take sufficient time to allow your self to think about what you want.

As my Grandma used to say, "Marry in haste, repent at leisure."

For a relationship to survive all these challenges a certain natural ease with each other is essential. If you have to persuade your partner to be involved in an interest with you, it is much harder than if you already share a passion for the same interest.

Not just a passion for sex but a passionate interest – for motorbikes, for ballroom dancing, gardening – whatever you truly chose as individuals. The passion may not necessarily be a 'doing' interest. It may be in the silent ease of 'being' together, each thoroughly enjoying the same moment. If you are passionate about watching a sunset and share this with someone who feels strongly too, there is a 'wow!' feeling.

The 'wow!' comes from 'I love it' and I see the same loving in my partner.

With all this in mind I suggested that Marianne and Joe take away a checklist and think about their next step. You may find it helpful to use the same checklist when you are 'in love' and think that the future together is looking good. Or answer from memory of when you were 'in love'.

Check these indicators and score one point for each yes answer.

Positive signals for continuing from 'in love'

Do you :
- feel respected
- feel listened to
- care about the other
- have interesting conversation
- have common interests, present before meeting each other
- have a similar sense of humour
- have a willingness to change
- share chores fairly
- find the other sexually attractive
- have pleasurable sex
- have a feeling of enchantment sometimes
- feel 'wow' together sometimes

Are you:
- aware that you have been on Cloud Nine
- aware that you know only a little about this person
- accepting of the way he/she is. (Rather than hoping he/she will change to what you want)
- willing to wait and see
- tolerant of the moods and attitudes of the other

Have you:
- met each other's friends and family

- talked about problems
- talked about your past
- discussed big issues, children, finance, where each wants to live, etc
- retained your own goals
- talked about what you like during sex

If you answered 'Yes' to:

0-6. Stop. Think very seriously about why you want to (or if you are thinking of your past – why you did) continue. Would it help you to talk to a counsellor about your reasons that make you need this relationship?

7-15. Caution. Think about the statements you said 'No' to. Can you talk about those now?

16-22. Go ahead. Always one step at a time as you explore sharing more with each other.

Ken Keyes in his, *The Power of Unconditional Love*,[13] states, 'Be aware that falling in love is not a basis for commitment.' This may shock you if you cling to the idea that love and marriage go together like a horse and carriage. The divorce rate of close to 50% is the real shock that should change your view when you are considering a long-term relationship.

You may delay formal marriage and try living together. But if you have already committed mentally to the permanence of the relationship you can fail to use this time to show each other who you really are and what you really want in life. Joe and Marianne had fallen into this trap.

If you are willing to fully reveal your true selves you will discover sooner rather than later whether you are compatible with your partner. Consider that in the first flush of romance you may have chosen the wrong partner – for you – and this may be why you are feeling uncomfortable. Had Marianne told Joe that she avoided the beach because she was easily sunburnt? Had Joe realised that she would not enjoy surfing, their relationship may have developed in a different way. Instead, they kept these (and other) differences under wraps. 'In love' they moved into the honeymoon suite.

Sharing a honeymoon without a marriage contract is no easier than being married though it does allow a less complicated separation if you decide you are not compatible. You may worry that without the bond of marriage it is too easy to abandon ship during rough weather. If you learn how to talk about and resolve problems, leaving over minor issues is less likely, married or not. The high divorce rate does not support that marriage itself helps two people resolve their problems.

If you have a sexual problem or even a misgiving about sex (or anything else!) when you are 'in love', you need to talk to your partner now. It does not get any easier later on. The longer you leave a problem the harder it becomes to discuss. You may hope that a problem will disappear by itself and it may. But it may not. Talking does not make things worse if you approach things with love and honesty. Talking with each other can resolve much. If you find this difficult there are helpful guidelines in Part Four.

Jane and Robert found it difficult to talk about their problem. They were pained to admit that sex was a problem right from the beginning of their relationship. The more time passed, the harder it became to tell to anyone else that they had not had sexual intercourse. Jane aged 28 was a university lecturer. Robert aged 35 was a nurse. Robert had been married before for three years and was divorced when they met six years ago. When they came to see me they had been happily married for four years. In this time they had moved beyond the 'in love' stage. Other than sex they scored high on the 'positive signals' scale.

"I thought Robert was attractive. I still do. I was embarrassed when we couldn't completely make love." Jane squeezed the life out of her fingers.

Robert clarified what Jane meant. "She tenses up when I try to penetrate with my penis. It is like hitting a solid wall. I don't want to hurt her by forcing anything," Robert said with great gentleness.

"I don't know why it happens. I want him to. We enjoy sex otherwise but we can't go the whole way." Jane told me this in her quiet almost childlike voice. "I'm embarrassed telling you. I doubt anyone else has let a problem go on for such a long time."

I wondered why they had waited so long though this is not as unusual as you may think. Many people wait years before seeking help with a sex problem. Sex is a private area and most hope they can sort things out on their own. But I soon understood why they had come along now.

"We've managed so far, but we have to do something. We want to start a family," Robert explained.

"We talk about everything and Robert has been so understanding," Jane told me with real affection for Robert, holding his hand as she spoke.

But Robert revealed his despondency. "I've tried for so long that I'm losing interest and half the time now I can't keep an erection."

Delay in dealing with their problem had made things worse. Robert had decreasing desire, which I thought resulted from his mind not motivating his penis to stay hard.

I heard how hard they had tried to overcome their problems. Jane struggled to relax and let things happen naturally but it did not work. Tightness in the muscles to the entrance of the vagina (called vaginismus) is generally related to emotional tension at the time of sex. In Jane, the cause of this tension was initially a mystery. It took many sessions to piece together the many reasons why this problem continued to occur. The clues came together bit by bit.

Jane twisted her fingers around and around. "When I was aged 9, I stayed with a friend overnight. Her father came into the bedroom and *touched her all over. Then he made me join in. Sometimes I get flashes of that when Robert and I are sexual."*

How frequently I have heard this anguish. Sexual abuse damages the development of healthy sexual feelings. There are, however, many variables as to how abuse is expressed in the individual. I am careful to place the impact of past sexual abuse in the context of the child's life then and their adult life in the present. I have found it insufficient, to fully resolve problems, to jump to the conclusion that sexual abuse is the only relevant cause of a problem.

"I couldn't tell anyone at the time, Mum was ill and I didn't want to be a trouble," came from a tiny voice.

It was the impact of her mother's illness and having no one to tell as well as the abuse that presented much unfinished business from Jane's childhood. Jane did talk about the abuse at length and was able to resolve this particular emotional wound. Sexual abuse is a complex issue that deserves fuller attention. (Should you seek extra help, there are some specific comments and information on local support groups, therapists and books in 'References'). But the vaginismus did not get any better. What continued to intrigue me was what made them tolerate their situation for six years. For any difficult situation to be so persistent, there are usually complex reasons. It transpired there certainly were and in Part Three when we consider updating childhood learning you will understand their situation better. Concerns originating in the past are commonly relevant to understanding the background to sex problems that can exist even when a couple are 'in love'.

You can ponder some of the factors from the past that might have contributed to the problems present for the couples you have read about in this section (or for your self):

- ଔ anxiety about commitment
- ଔ anxiety of talking openly to partner

- previous sexual abuse
- inadequate sex education
- anxiety about sexual performance
- unfinished business related to family of origin
- religious views with sex as sin
- guilt over divorce or death of a previous partner
- physical or mental illness
- the choice of the wrong partner – for you
- the burden on a partner of unfulfilled needs

This covers a wide area of possible factors and there may be others. If a problem persists you can appreciate that professional counselling may be valuable at this time.

At a more worrying level some warning bells should go off, alarming you to serious dysfunctional behaviour when 'in love'. Alcohol abuse, violence and gambling are extremes. They are not usually present 'in love' because the good feelings generated remove the need for addictive behaviour. If such behaviour exists early on, a serious problem is present. Either abandon ship now or if you want to stay, seek professional help before even considering a long-term relationship.

*I need someone's hands
To lead me through the night.
I need someone's arms
To squeeze and hold me tight.
And when the night begins
and I'm at an end
You know I need your love so bad.*

                    'Need Your Love So Bad'
                        Little Willie John

Chapter Eight

Fog warning

In the honeymoon suite the mist that swirls around seems romantic. Then you hear a fog warning and the mist becomes more sinister. You begin to wonder about the safety of the love boat. Is it constructed strongly from shared love or from the less durable need for the relationship? The two are not the same.

Need is based on fear of scarcity (you do not already have enough or there is a shortage) of what you desire. Sharing the abundance of what you already have in your own heart with a companion or sex partner is love without demand. This is a difficult concept particularly if you have not recognised the difference between needing and sharing before.

You can start by asking your self, "Have I ever fallen 'in love' to get my needs met?" There are many reasons for needing a relationship. Check to see if you had (or have) a relationship because you needed:

- an ego boost
- the 'high'
- attention
- love
- financial support

- someone to help you get over your previous relationship
- a housekeeper/handyman
- a second parent for your child/children
- cheering up
- a sex partner
- a companion
- to take care of someone (needing to be needed)
- to meet the expectations of society/peer group/ family

As you read this you may ask what is wrong with wanting what is on the list. The problem is not the wanting but the **needing** of any of these. If you want to share something on this list with another, that is the icing on the cake. If you **need** a partner to provide it you don't have a cake on which to put the icing!

Needing is very different from desiring to share the love you have with someone else. Need places an expectation on the other. This unspoken burden can lead to the downfall of the long-term success of the relationship. But it takes the completion of much unfinished business from childhood to be able to distinguish needing a relationship from sharing love. Some examples of the difference between sharing and needing will make this clearer.

1. *An ego boost*

Joe was blonde and tall with strong muscles and Marianne had been attracted by his body.

"I felt a million dollars when my friends admired Joe's good looks."

Marianne needed Joe to be handsome to help her feel good.

"My last boyfriend teased me about my breasts. He suggested I have breast implants to make them bigger. I thought about it a lot. But I didn't have enough money. Joe told me I was beautiful just the way I was."

Marianne was very unsure of her own attractiveness. She was caught in the modern cult of the body beautiful. Marianne needed Joe to reassure her that she was desirable.

Laura Esquivel in her delightful novel, The Law of Love,[14] has a guardian angel talk about the role of ego in choosing a partner.

> *A person with an ego problem will want as a partner someone who is a prized and valuable object. The most handsome or beautiful, the most intelligent, and so on... The partner thereby confers status and evokes admiration... The perfect partner could have walked right by the egoist without provoking a second look, because he did not possess an observable talent or muscles... The voice of the ego urges him to choose someone not meant for him.*

Wise words from a guardian angel who in the story is trying to help his charge choose a compatible partner.

Looking for someone to fulfil your needs is common. Even therapists have done it (hopefully in their past) and learned by this.

2. The 'high'

I recall being 28 years old. Working as a general medical practitioner. I thought my life was boring. I needed a 'high'.

> *"I was full of the excitement of a sailing holiday around Corsica when I collided with Mario. He was also sailing with a group of friends. I was instantly impressed. A suntanned body to die for. I thought he was Adonis. In broken English we found we had everything in common. A candlelit dinner overlooking the picturesque harbour of Porto Fino and I had 'fallen'. We sailed separately each day but each evening I waited for his white boat to come alongside. 'High? 'I was up Everest. Our romance fluoresced.*

"We returned to our own countries and kept in expectant contact. Our next meeting was in Paris. Entwined, we made love, dined, gazed at the Impressionist paintings. We walked the whole of Paris in each other's arms. I savoured every luscious moment. Back in dull England more fervent correspondence and telephone calls led to my flying to Italy to ski with Mario. I remember sending him a photograph after the holiday. I wrote the loving inscription, 'Two people on top of the world'.

"Mario visited me in England. We toured the glorious countryside. We nestled beside open fires in country pubs. When he left we were both bereft. No longer could we live apart. Within three months I joined him. I found a stressed, businessman who worked long hours, a foreign culture and no one to share a joke with in my own language. He also had a difficult ex-wife. I left a few weeks later."

I realised then that if my life on my own became more interesting I would not need to find a high in romance. Next time I wanted a 'high' I tried abseiling – it was less risky.

3. Attention

Peter had been having an affair. When Judy found out she threatened to leave. Instead they came for counselling.

"Judy used to be so thoughtful when we were dating. She kept my favourite beer in the fridge. She always had time for me no matter how busy she was. I could drop by her place anytime and she would always stop what she was doing. If she had made arrangements to see friends she would cancel with them if I invited her out. That's how much she loved me. It was wonderful when we were first married. But since she had the baby she has no time for me. I feel completely unwanted. She's not even interested in sex. No wonder I had an affair."

Peter came from a family of seven children. With so many in the family he had jostled for attention, but of course, there was never enough. Judy took care of his ravenous need for attention. Until the baby also needed attention. This change was a challenge for them both.

4. *Financial support*
Cheryl had been used to a good standard of living. She had been raised on a wealthy farm and attended an exclusive school. She came to see me after her fourth major relationship exploded in spectacular fashion.

"I married Julian, a partner in a highly successful law firm. We had two children. I was a perfect hostess and we prospered. It was OK at first. As time went on there were many reasons we were not happy. Julian made some stupid share dealings and most of our money was gone. After 18 years of marriage we divorced. After the divorce I lived in an awful financial mess. I met other men of course. I was very attracted to men who were successful. I admired them, but they all turned out to be disasters."

Cheryl admired wealthy men but had never admired herself. She had creative talents that she had only ever explored as a minor hobby. She had never had the confidence to explore taking care of her own financial needs by turning her hobby into a career. Cheryl needed a man to support her financially.

During therapy she found the confidence to start her own business and to care for herself. She became free to choose a partner independent of his ability to be a provider of financial support.

5. *Someone to help you get over your previous relationship*
6. *A housekeeper*
7. *A second parent for your child/children*
If this sounds like an irresistible combination consider George. George had been married previously for 12 years when his first wife, Wendy, left him. He came when his second marriage, to Anne, was on the rocks.

"I was devastated when my wife left. Three months later I met Anne. She had been separated for six months. She was everything my wife was not. Anne cooked wonderful dinners. She went to the football with me. She really cared for my three young boys when they visited. Anne had three older children of her own. She had great problems with disciplining them without her husband. I was a good father to them."

Of course there was more George had to say but in this short declaration much was revealed. George and Anne needed each other. Neither had learned to care for their own needs before they met. They had not allowed themselves any time to do so. Instead, each found the other in need. This relationship that developed was closer to a mother/son and father/daughter relationship than one of equal sharing.

8. Cheering up

Neal was sad when he told me of his lost love, Helen. He told me before he met her he had been feeling miserable. His job was not going well. He was having difficulties with his boss. He had lost hope of the promotion he wanted. His social life was poor. Many evenings he sat at home watching television. If he went out, he went to a club to have a few beers to drown his sorrows.

"At the Christmas party at work I met Helen. She was older than me. She said how sad I looked. She offered to cheer me up and told some terrific jokes. I laughed for the first time in months."

This was just what Neal needed. In the following months they had many dates.

At first Helen was flattered by the constant attention that Neal paid her, but eventually felt pursued by this same attention and called a halt to the relationship. Neal continued to 'phone, write and send flowers. He wanted to recapture the person who fulfilled his need to feel happy.

9. A sex partner
10. A companion
11. Love

This was Lorraine's favourite combination when she was looking for a partner (when she needed a partner!) Lorraine met Russell when she first moved to Melbourne. She did not know many people. She was lonely.

"I spotted an attractive man buying the same newspaper as myself. We smiled. Next day I was at the newspaper shop at the same time and spent half an hour browsing through the magazines. My wait was worthwhile. In strode Russell. This time we talked. He had recently moved from Sydney. Like me Russell didn't know anyone. I felt magnetised. We 'bumped into each other' the next day and the romance began. We had many similar interests; great sex, and he told me he loved me (all in the first week.) I was swept off my feet. Russell had met all my needs. That great romance lasted six weeks."

Lorraine's own commentary illustrates how needy she was when she met Russell and vice versa. Their neediness swamped each other and led to a hot, but brief relationship.

12. To take care of someone

Geraldine was a 'good wife and mother'. Her husband, Tim, had his own successful business.

"Tim works hard. We have just built a beautiful new house. But somehow I feel confined, like I want to scream. These days I don't want to make love with Tim but I feel I should. He's done nothing wrong. He's a good man. All my married life I've cared for Tim and the children. I like to make life easier for Tim. I lay out his clothes each morning, make sure he eats breakfast, and pack a lunch for him, as he's often too busy to get anything for himself. I organise the home, holidays, every-

thing. I try to anticipate what Tim needs and make sure it is done."

Geraldine was so busy caring for everyone else she forgot to care for herself. She put all her energy into others, in the hope she would be needed and loved in return. Of course she was. But that did not quench her inner thirst to be loved for who she was, not just the care she provided. Needing to be needed limited Geraldine to always providing what she thought Tim wanted. It restricted Tim as he felt obliged to appreciate everything Geraldine did for him, whether he wanted it done or not. They were both exhausted by this burden.

13. *To meet the expectations of society/peer group/family*

Nick needed to please his family. He managed his father's three Greek restaurants. He was an important member of the family business.

"From the age of 30 my father was always asking when was I going to get married. He and Mama invited daughters of their friends to dinner – often. We were catering for a huge crowd one night when I saw Anthi. I thought she was spectacular. Unfortunately, my father spotted her too. He virtually pushed us together. I didn't really mind because I wanted to meet her.

"We started to date. My parents joked about a wedding – soon. I liked Anthi but I wasn't sure if I wanted to marry her. But my parents were sure.

"'She's a beautiful girl. She's crazy about you. What are you waiting for? You'll be too old to enjoy children. It would make us so happy,' was all I heard from my parents.

"In the end I thought they were right. I proposed and Anthi accepted. Our parents made the wedding plans. There were 400 guests, with the works. It became a nightmare. All the talk was about the wedding and grandchildren to take over the business. Anthi and I hardly had a chance to catch our breaths.

"We got married and it was a beautiful wedding. But..."

They came to talk to me about the 'but...' that had occurred since the wedding. Nick had been rushed along trying to meet the expectations of his parents.

There is cultural pressure to have a partner in many societies to be socially accepted. This can lead people to sacrifice their self for the sake of having a relationship. Often parents who gave up their own identities for the sake of marriage expect the same of their children. Their culture was obsessed by the value of the relationship itself, rather than the value of love and respect of their own self and each other. Many struggled with the resentment this caused. You now have more choice but such choice can be confusing. Beware of making your choice to please others. Someone else's needs are the hardest of all to meet.

All these needs are common. To understand neediness, go back to your childhood learning. Neediness is perfectly reasonable for a dependent child. When you are little you do need someone else to take care of you. A child should continue to develop to become a completely independent adult, able to take care of your own needs. But few people leave home as fully mature individuals.

In your early years you develop insecurities. Big or small, they become the basis of your needs. One day, for your own peace of mind you have to face insecurities, doubts and fears for yourself. In doing so you become relieved of need and can open fully to love.

Remember Marianne? One of her sensitive areas was her appearance. When her last boyfriend told her that her breasts were too small, she was hurt. Unsure of her self worth, she still needed to be told she was beautiful. She had needed this as a child but had never heard it enough to settle her fear that she was not beautiful (and therefore loveable). Joe told her she was beautiful and she felt good that she could attract a handsome man. She felt reassured by Joe. The problem is that someone else can never reassure you enough to overcome your own insecurities.

Marianne had to learn that her beauty lay inside her, not in her surface looks. She needed to reassess her doubts remaining from childhood. If she could update this learning, she would not need anyone else to tell her she was beautiful. Marianne would know for herself. Realising that her last boyfriend did not like her breast size he could find himself another woman. She could choose a man not to satisfy her need for an ego boost but to share love with him.

How do you tell the difference between needing and sharing? Try listening to your self-talk.

Do you say to your self statements that sound like needing?

- It is essential that you do this for me.
- It is the only way I can be happy.
- I can't do it for myself.
- If you don't give me what I need I'll keep on demanding (or I'll look for someone else).
- You should say 'Yes' to taking care of my need.

Or sound as though you are sharing?

- I would enjoy sharing this with you.
- It isn't essential that you do.
- If you don't I can manage myself.
- It's fine for you to choose 'Yes' or 'No' when I say what I want.

Neediness is a pain when you are an adult – if you expect someone else to take care of your need. You can grow beyond need. You can begin this process by identifying your needs.

Write down your needs – the ones that you hope someone else will take care of for you. You can use the list above as a starter to recognise your needs. But there are many others.

I recall a relatively small need from my own list that became a challenge. I used to need someone else to talk to difficult tradesmen for me. I would put off talking to them about my complaint. I could not stand it when they became angry. But by learning not to be intimidated by anger I can now stand it. It will never be my favourite pastime but I can do it. We all have these areas we prefer to avoid but relying on someone else can make you needy and dependent on their support.

With your list of needs in mind you have a basis from which to think back and recall when and why they began. This can be difficult to do but the needy clients described were able to look back to their early years and make the connection between their present needs and the past.

With some help they recognised they had these needs most of their life. Some were able to shift from needing to sharing in their relationships by taking responsibility for their own needs and not expecting their partner to do this.

These thoughts are just as applicable to sex as they are to anything else. Of course, it takes two people to have sexual intercourse but sex flows more tenderly from sharing rather than need. This becomes possible as your relationship continues to grow and mature. This progress is clearly seen in one of the couples, Greg and Pauline, who join us in Chapter Nine.

If you have chosen someone because they take care of one (or more) of your needs do not be hard on your self. You are normal. Growing to become a fully independent person takes many years after you first call your self an adult. Children use the term 'grown ups' for people over the age of 21, but most of us are not completely 'grown up' for many years after that.

Much depends on the challenges that life presents you to grow up in the areas that remain limited by doubts and fears. Your voyage aboard the love boat challenges you to face any insecurities that lurk in your depths. Changing from neediness to personal responsibility for your self is part of the maturing process that is required to stay afloat during troubled waters.

∼

Part Three

Troubled Waters

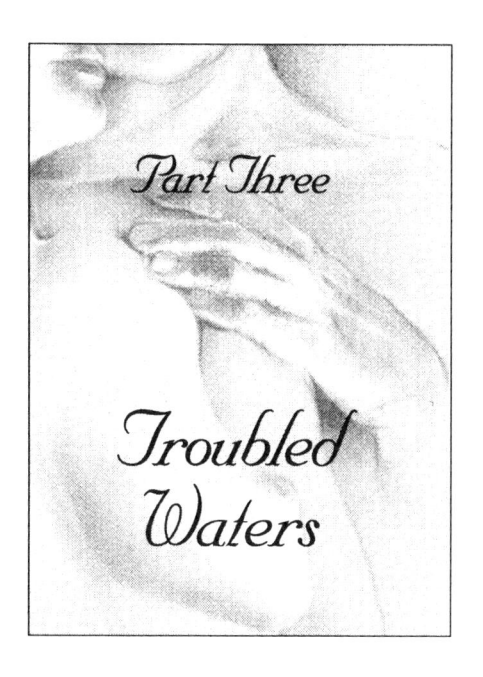

The course of true love never did run smooth.

'Midsummer Night's Dream'
William Shakespeare

When your heart's on fire
You must realise
Smoke gets in your eyes.

'Smoke Gets in Your Eyes'
The Platters

Chapter Nine

Out of the mist

*E*ventually the realities of life intrude rudely upon your stay in the honeymoon suite. Work, chores, loan repayments, ambition, in-laws, pregnancy and children insist on being noticed. They force you to step out of the mist to explore the rest of the love boat and continue on your voyage.

Beyond the mist you see with 20:20 vision you see not only the good in your partner but also the bad and the ugly. You find your self under the microscope also. This can come as a shock. You were convinced that you knew everything about your beloved. You may have known everything you wanted to know, but not everything there is to know. The things you do not like about each other come into sharp focus.

You may be horrified to notice your partner's previously amusing habits drive you nuts. He clips his toenails into the carpet. Her long hairs block the shower outflow. Or more disturbing behaviour is seen. He gets angry and yells when you want to talk about his job. She sulks and will not talk at all, when you want to, about money. How could you have been so blind?

You may wonder what is wrong. There is nothing wrong. Simply the honeymoon period is over. This is the part that Hollywood has not prepared you for. Scriptwriters instead concentrate on a few dramatic options suited only to a world of fantasy:

1. They kill off one or both partners ('Titanic', 'Romeo and Juliet', 'Love Story'). This leaves the remaining partner and the audience, grieving for the loss of 'perfect' love.

2. They leave the couple soon after the most romantic wedding, fading into the sunset, to live supposedly happily ever after. ('Cinderella', 'Man from Snowy River').

3. Hollywood scriptwriters make the couple so rich that they can continue endless romantic dinners and exotic holidays. This plot also requires they have infrequent time together so they can continue their 'in love' dream. They never have time to enter the reality of most couples.

Opening your eyes to the full knowledge of your partner can be hard to bear. You may not know what to do next. You may be convinced you have limited choices because you feel cemented into the relationship. But you always have choice though deciding what to do can be more challenging than Hollywood dares to imagine.

Compatibility

What do you do once you hit the reality of troubled waters? A starting point is to consider your compatibility with the person you stepped on board the love boat with. Do you still want to share the voyage? You embarked in Provisional Love knowing only very little about each other but thinking you knew everything.

If you accept the challenge of this essential phase in a relationship, you can make a start by finding out if you have sufficient areas of compatibility to choose to remain together. It is natural to be disappointed that your partner is not perfect. Do you want this real person? Facing the reality of who you are and who your partner is helps you to decide. It works better than subduing your concerns.

Out of the mist Marianne and Joe needed to do this. Joe had answered the questions on the checklist, 'Positive signals for continuing, from 'in love' (p.98). He had scored 8. Marianne said she had forgotten to read the questionnaire.

> "We don't seem to have many interests in common. I want Marianne to come surfing with me. I love surfing. She used to come with me but now she hangs around the house most of her spare time. We talk about what we've done at work each day. That's about all there is now."

Joe's eyes rolled to the heavens. Joe and Marianne were feeling that somehow they had failed when everyone else had not. However, the truth is such disillusionment is common. They would have been better prepared for this if society would be truthful about real relationships. It would help if we stopped filling people's heads with romantic 'happily ever after' expectations. Continuing a long-term relationship takes some special ingredients. Love is only one of these.

Joe and Marianne had to face their reality. They had major differences and did not seem to have much in common. The novelty of the relationship was wearing thin. Rather than face their differences they now spent little time together. They hoped the holiday would return them to mists of the honeymoon suite. The intense proximity had the opposite effect and brought things to a head.

> Joe continued: "I want to spend some time surfing in Bali one day but Marianne wants to settle down and buy a house together. I love Marianne but I don't know what to do. If we could sort out this sex thing I'm sure things would be better."
>
> Marianne replied: "I love Joe. I changed jobs and everything to be with him. I don't understand what is happening to us. We still have sex sometimes and that feels nice but I wish he didn't 'come' so quickly. He gets satisfied but I don't."

I suspected that in this Marianne was wrong. Joe had plenty of orgasms but was not fully satisfied. Sex was not bringing him joy. Marianne's desire for sex was also waning, not because of premature ejaculation but due to the confusion of feelings that were emerging for her.

It was time for Marianne and Joe to take a really honest look at each other and inside themselves. Why was each of them staying in this relationship? Did they need the relationship rather than having a good basis for sharing love? Marianne needed Joe to boost her ego. Joe needed a sex partner and a companion. Their needs had become a burden on each other in the absence of compatibility.

"I don't want to have to keep saying she's beautiful. I think she is, but I feel stupid to keep saying it."

"It used to feel good when you did," Marianne sighed.

"It used to feel good when you wanted to come surfing with me, it was good when you wanted sex - but they don't happen now either." Joe's voice had a sharp edge.

I was not hearing the conversation of two people 'in love'. They were 'in reality'. But 'in love' they had made a commitment - before they knew each other. Marianne had changed her job and left her own apartment to live with Joe. Now things were not going well and this caused distress for them both.

Sex had little chance to improve in this situation. I knew it was not the appropriate time to consider the premature ejaculation. They needed to resolve whether they both felt they had enough, beyond 'in love', to share the voyage on the love boat. I urged them to deal with the cause of their problem not the end result.

Separating

Joe and Marianne returned to Sydney after their holidays, still confused but ready to talk. Marianne 'phoned me a few weeks later:

"Joe and I talked a lot after seeing you. It was hard but in the end Joe decided to go to Bali for a few months. I didn't want to go. I have a good job here. I was upset when he left. I missed him at first. Now I think it is for the best. I'm spending time with my friends. We go ice-skating, maybe I'll meet someone at skating. I loved Joe but I do realise that 'in love' we didn't know each other very well. But I'll go slower next time. I want to sort out a few of my own problems in the meantime. I'd like to get rid of my hang up about my looks. I'm working on it! Thanks, talking helped me see that Joe and I had totally different views on life."

Marianne and Joe's dilemma was typical of the stage after 'in love'. Their individual differences not noticed, or ignored earlier, had begun to emerge. If you have been in a similar situation you may also have hoped that the other would change to be more the way you wanted (preferably similar to you), as Joe and Marianne had. Eventually Marianne and Joe realised they were not well suited even though they had strong feelings for each other. They recognised they were not compatible and decided to part.

It was important that they were clear about why they reached this decision. They needed each other for an ego boost and had rushed helter skelter into commitment. On the plus side their relationship had offered them the opportunity to look at their patterns of behaviour so they may now approach a new relationship in a better way. What they learned would help them both avoid repeating such a painful experience.

It would have been easy to view their sexual problem as the cause of their separating. But then Joe would have been stuck trying to find a cure for his 'premature ejaculation' and Marianne would have been looking for a man who was slower in bed. Instead, they were able to recognise their differences and allow that the differences were not ones they wanted to accept. Marianne also developed an awareness of some of her neediness that hooked her onto Joe so quickly. There was a dependency in her love. Their love was provisional. It turned out not to be the basis of a long-term relationship. There was no reason to expect it should be. You learn the joys of loving through a tortuous process, however much you might desire it to be otherwise.

Joe contacted me many months later. He had spent time in Bali surfing and pursuing Eros.

"I had a few flings in Bali. It was easy to have sex. I had no problems with premature ejaculation. Sex was casual and was fun. And before you freak out Doc, I did use condoms.

"When I returned to Sydney, I met a really nice girl, Joanne. I can't believe it, but I had the same problem, premature ejaculation, with her. I read about where you can squeeze below the knob of the penis just before coming, to try to slow down. It didn't work for me though. I tried to think of something else to distract myself but then I didn't enjoy sex much. Then I thought about what you'd said was the cause of the problem. I decided to back off a bit and see what happened. Gradually sex is getting better. Jo and I get on very well and there's no pressure. I realised that she is in no hurry to settle down. That feels good."

At first Joe had not believed that the anxiety of rushing into a relationship contributed to his problem. Eros can be such a strong drive that compatibility gets overlooked as attention is focused on successful sex.

From this viewpoint Joe thought he would simply find a technique to solve his problem. He tried the common techniques suggested for premature ejaculation. He distracted his mind as his excitement and arousal mounted rather than allow the moment of orgasm to come when it will. He tried boring thoughts to slow down or stop ejaculation. He had not enjoyed that much nor the squeeze technique. Finally, he realised the best technique was talking.

When he talked with Joanne he discovered she did not want to rush any commitment and thought that some space was good for them both. They did not move in together. They continued to maintain 'separate cabins' and each pursued different activities as well as sharing their passion of surfing. They allowed time to discuss their past and hopes for the future. They opted for the slow process of getting to know each other before booking a 'shared berth'.

Staying longer

Joe and Marianne had good reasons to separate. But what if you have good reasons to continue the relationship? You feel 'love' for your partner (do you need to go back to Chapter Six to review what type of love you are experiencing?) but do you like your partner? What can you do to work things out? How do you handle the differences that arise between you? If you are not going to leave, how do you deal with staying?

Reversing

You may direct your energy into returning to the sanctuary of the honeymoon suite by recreating romantic episodes. But somehow they do not feel the same as when you were 'in love'. They may feel more like a struggle than a pleasurable effort and offer only a temporary respite before you are tossed again back into troubled waters. You cannot avoid the challenges of a love relationship by going backwards.

Getting stuck

You may run aground and decide the easiest option is to bury your head in the sand. The constant joy of being 'in love' begins to wane as you discover the person you were sure was right for you is not perfect after all. You may find some ways to distract your self from this uncomfortable truth.

In the ostrich position it is easy to find other things to occupy your mind. Time consuming activities - work, TV, computers, children, hobbies, an affair, food, alcohol or other drugs can become a substitute. Are you doing these for the pleasure they bring or because you need to distract your mind? Distractions may offer temporary relief from your swelling panic. Unfortunately, while you are busy ignoring the real issues a storm is brewing. If you leave problems until you can no longer stand them, you are likely to leave each other.

The relationship is no longer hearts and roses. You are uncomfortable sometimes. You are fed up sometimes. When you try to talk you end up in a mess. Nothing gets resolved. Perhaps the way you have been trying to solve problems needs a review.

Disillusionment will often result in conflict. Unfortunately, at this stage of a relationship you may only have win/lose conflict models on which to fall back for guidance. Families, politicians and armies commonly use this style. It is part of our culture. What 'rules' do you follow in win/lose conflict and where do they lead you?

The basics of win/lose

Rules

- attack/defend
- closed minds
- blame
- do not listen fully
- have expectations of the other
- "you should..."
- do not try to understand the opposite view
- try to get the other to agree with you
- do not reveal all you feel
- try to end discussion as soon as possible

Results
- confusion
- anger
- argument
- withdrawal
- at least one person feels bad
- unpalatable resolution of problem
- frustration
- winner and a loser

Resolutions
- give in
- walk away
- unhealthy compromise with a heavy heart
- violence
- repeated arguments
- topic becomes taboo
- future avoidance of conflict (using more distractions)

Win/lose conflict is not just expressed in words and feelings; it flows through your heart to the sexual arena. If you cannot resolve problems by your attempts to talk you may accept being stuck and search for distractions instead. Eventually the disappointment that you feel in sex that does not satisfy your inner desires becomes hard to ignore. This was the point that Greg and Pauline had reached when they came to discuss their problems. Their conflict was obvious, as it was open and vocal.

Open conflict

Pauline, aged 36, and Greg, aged 42, came to see me because every time their love boat was buffeted by storms the only response they could make was to fight about whose fault it was. They were in troubled waters. They had been married for 16 years. They had a son aged 15 and a daughter aged 12. They came at a time when their arguments were focused on sex.

"*The problem is she doesn't like sex,*" Greg began.

Pauline disagreed. "*I do, but not as often as you. You want it all the time.*"

Their view of the problem was clearly different. It sounded as though each thought the other was at fault. It was easy to see how an argument could rapidly develop. I asked what they had tried so far to sort out this problem. Greg was quick to defend himself to show the effort that he had made.

"*I have tried everything. Romantic dinners, presents, 'blue' movies, not asking for sex - hoping she would, the lot. She is just not interested.*"

"*I've tried too,*" said Pauline. "*He gets frustrated about not having sex. I realise how tense he is. He works hard for the kids and I. He's a great provider.*

"*In the end I have sex to please him. He calms down and is lovely. But a couple of days later it's the same all over again. I can't do it any more.*" *Pauline's mouth set in a hard line.*

"*I have no choice about work,*" *Greg countered.* "*It costs a lot to live and put the kids through school. I run my own business and put in long hours. When I come home I'm stressed out. I see my lovely wife, I want to make love and feel the release from the heavy day. If she loved me she'd want to as well,*" *he added sharply.*

Pauline hastily returned to soothing. This was her pattern of responding to the tension she detected in Greg's voice.

"*But I get tired too. The kids aren't easy. I'm studying part time so that soon I can get a job and help out.*"

"*But you lie around watching TV until all hours.*" *Greg slammed home his annoyance.* "*I want you to come to bed when I do. Then we* could relax and make love. You just don't want me." Pauline winced at his words.

Greg genuinely thought he had tried everything. He had tried everything that he knew. His desperation to find a solution was shrouded in his annoyance and frustration. His only way of avoiding the non-sexual issues that secretly worried him was to maintain his conviction that Pauline was simply not interested in sex. The possibilities for discussion were limited by his focus.

In fact, both Greg and Pauline were using sex to relieve their different stresses. For Greg his stress was excessive work. He was also stressed by his overwhelming need to be reassured that he and Pauline had no other problems. Both these contributed to his avoidance of resolving the differences between them.

Pauline had sex to relieve the pressure from Greg. Rather than deal with their problems Pauline opted for the distraction of television. She was also busy with children and study. Greg believed that love meant Pauline should do something to please him even when she did not want to. Thus, he pressed for sex, needing Pauline to prove her love in this way. Because he needed more she wanted less. Unfortunately, sex then contributed to their growing resentments. Rather than soothe their stress it made things worse.

Sex was just one way that Greg and Pauline played out their conflicts. It failed to resolve their problems but the focus on sex did deflect their attention from what they did not want to acknowledge. They had many differences and had not found a satisfactory way to discuss these.

To shift the focus I asked if they argued about other things.

"Not really," Greg quickly replied.

"Well there was the weekend," Pauline tentatively offered.

"But that was nothing much," shrugged Greg. "After all we made up afterwards."

Even if it did seem like nothing I very much wanted to hear about it. A great deal can be learned listening to two people discuss their differences, even minor ones. With a little persuasion Pauline continued.

"*Well, the garden is a mess and Greg didn't want to help out and we had a row.*"

"*Now hang on. I started out really politely.*" Greg's face reddened.

I asked them to try and recall as closely as possible what they said and how they said it.

"*Well I asked her really nicely, 'What would you like to do this weekend?' I said.*"

I asked them to continue in the present tense, as though the events were happening right at this moment. I find it helps to recapture the feelings as well as the words.

"*Well you know the garden is a mess. I think we should clear it up,*" Pauline cajoled.

"*The garden isn't too bad. Wouldn't you like to do something else?*" Greg replied.

Greg had wanted to go fishing and hoped Pauline would come along. Pauline was expecting Greg to do the garden. She hoped he would do something to please her. After all if he wanted her to do things for him, like sex, he should do the garden. Maybe if Greg had done the garden, Pauline would have given him sex. But then they both would have been playing with sex as a bargaining tool.

From the beginning I could see their style of talking was a tangle of unstated hopes. Greg began by asking Pauline what she wanted to do, rather than say what he would like. He would have liked to please Pauline, but he was also keen to go fishing. But he did not say so. He had hoped she would read his mind and suggest they go to the river, then he could fish.

Pauline, in fact, wanted to catch up on some study and she wanted to see the garden tidy. She tried to get some of what she wanted by telling Greg what they **should** do. The word should often triggers guilt. It is usually a double whammy as both partners become burdened with should. Having started with what Greg should do, Pauline felt it would be selfish to say what she wanted.

Greg tried to steer Pauline away from the should by telling her that in his view the garden was not too bad. Pauline then thought he was saying that her view of the garden being a mess was exaggerated and wrong. She felt hurt and annoyed. Pauline responded with her own method of defense. She subtly entered attack mode.

"*I've been asking you to help for weeks. You keep putting it off,*" Pauline whined.

"*You're so boring. You used to like some fun, now all you want to do is stay at home.*" Greg became louder.

Now Greg felt annoyed and hurt. He went into attack mode also. Pauline knew Greg was angry. She hated conflict and wanted to settle things down. She also felt some fear that his anger might explode and, just like her father, he would break something. She returned to soothing Greg's ruffled feathers.

"*We don't have any spare money to go out,*" Pauline said softly.

"*That's not my fault. I work my butt off for you and the kids. You always remind me that I don't do enough,*" Greg shouted.

"I didn't say that!"

"*Sounded like that to me. I'm not staying here to listen to your nagging!*"

Greg maintained his anger. He had stormed out of the house slamming the door. The deterioration of their communication led to Greg think Pauline was blaming him for limited money. He felt unappreciated at that moment but extended that to all situations by saying always.

One occasion became added to his mental list. This added up to an all-encompassing resentment.

Greg was secretly worried that he was not earning enough money to support his family. Rather than discuss that particular problem, which hurt his male pride, Greg projected his own concerns about their limited finances back onto Pauline. He made it sound as though she blamed him. Pauline was secretly concerned that she was not contributing to the family income and that Greg was stressed about money. She was aware of his hurt when they had tried to discuss money in the past. It seemed easier to bury this important topic.

By this time the discussion was far away from the original point of what each wanted to do for the day. The unresolved problem of money had surfaced. Problems keep being regurgitated if they have not been sufficiently worked through. A respectful discussion with a view to a settlement needs to be had before the subject can be laid to rest. But like many of us, Pauline and Greg did not know how to do this.

Greg had gone fishing for the rest of the day but instead of a peaceful pleasure he had snagged his line in his impatience. Pauline had been angry too. She had felt a knot in her stomach as she fought her way through the garden. They both had a miserable day.

When Greg came home later in the afternoon he was ready to 'patch things up'.

"The garden looks nice," Greg began.

"Hmmph!" Greg tried to give Pauline a kiss. She turned her face away.

"You could say you're sorry." Pauline folded her arms across her chest.

"I'm sorry. Come on give me a kiss," Greg pleaded.

Greg started to touch Pauline's breasts to show he wanted everything to be alright between them.

"Don't, I'm tired." Pauline drew her mouth tight.

"You never want sex. I said I'm sorry."

Pauline knew he was sorry. She was weary from arguing and doing the garden. She did not really feel like sex. Not only was she tired but she felt that yet again a problem had taken them round in a circle. She also wanted everything to be alright. With a heavy heart she did what she thought was best and they had sex.

I asked what was sex like on that occasion. Greg contributed, 'fine.' I heard an 'OK' from Pauline. I asked them to talk more openly about their feelings at the time.

"I wish he hadn't flown off in a temper. It would have been good for once to sort things out. I didn't have any real desire for sex. I would have liked to talked some more and maybe just had a cuddle. It felt like we just keep going over the same problems again and again and never get anywhere."

"There you see she just wants a cuddle. She isn't interested in sex," snorted Greg.

I could see they were both trapped by their pain. Greg blamed Pauline. He knew only one solution to regain warmth between them — by having sex.

Pauline had gone along with him to regain peace. Neither had been willing to sort out the real problems. Both, however, had a part that wanted to find a better way but it was always defeated by the other part, which thought any further discussion would be a waste of time.

I asked again how each felt that evening during and after sex.

After considerable silence Greg sighed. "I felt lonely, she just lay there."

With tears in her eyes Pauline responded, "I felt lousy. It felt like rape."

Each had finally admitted to their own distress. They had also opened their hearts in this moment to hear each other's pain.

What messed up the communication between Pauline and Greg on this occasion? If you put your self into their places you may recognise what you, or your partner, have done in a similar situation.

In resorting to open conflict have you:
- blamed the other?
- had a fixed mind?
- tried to please the other by sacrificing your own desires?
- been stressed?
- found distractions to avoid dealing with a problem, e.g., TV, excessive work?
- not been open to accepting your partner's view as right for them?
- expected a partner to read your mind?
- had an expectation of how your partner should be?
- not acknowledged your own concerns, but projected them as coming from your partner?
- not shared how you felt?
- translated one occasion to 'always'?
- acted out of anger?
- become violent?

Arguments are not about resolution, they are about winning. 'In love' there is not the same need to win because you appear to find agreement on most things. As time passes your partner begins to say what they do not like about you. The way you relate changes in response. If you can not discuss the emerging differences with respect, eventually it becomes sink or swim.

Not one of these responses steers the love boat through a problem to reach new understanding. You will continue to be tossed from one storm through unnatural calm onto the next if you stay on the same course.

Finally, Pauline and Greg recognised not only their own pain but also felt the sadness of the other. It was the catalyst to consider new ways to tackle their problems. They could close off to each other yet again or be willing to try 'charting new waters', albeit with trepidation. Their next visit was a turning point for them.

∼

*It isn't that they can't see the solution.
It is that they can't see the problem.*

> G. K. Chesterton

Chapter Ten

All at sea

Greg and Pauline fought their storms out on the open deck but do you sit dining at the captain's table while the love boat is swamped with water? When the boat tilts precariously do you or your partner look the other way? On the surface you may appear to have achieved harmony, because you do not argue. But have you slipped into hidden conflict in which issues are avoided? Do you tolerate your differences with a combination of distractions, compromise and withdrawal?

On the surface do you continue to share the honeymoon suite by evading what makes you uncomfortable, but inside are you feeling 'all at sea'?

Do you stay together but apart?

This was the situation for Elaine and Roger. Roger, aged 49, taught art at high school. Elaine was 45. She helped Roger in his extra business in multi-level marketing of home products. They had a daughter aged 18 and a son aged 21 who lived away from home attending university. Elaine and Roger had lost their main distraction of children and were faced with only each other across the breakfast table.

Elaine attended on her own. She did not want to talk in the presence of her husband; in fact, she found it hard to talk at all.

"Things were alright. We managed. I never enjoyed sex but now I can't even bear him to touch me. I feel stupid because I love him. He's been so understanding. But now I find out he's had an affair. Oh no!"

Elaine disintegrated into sobs. I passed the tissues and gave her time to settle. Elaine had focused attention on their unsatisfactory sex life. I wondered how they had coped during their 24 years of marriage.

"On Sunday morning Roger closes the bedroom door. It's become a ritual and we have sex. I love him so I do it. Roger is very tender. He's very understanding. But recently I told him I just couldn't do it anymore. We've hardly spoken since."

This was obviously such a painful time for Elaine. Yet it was important that she talk to someone.

"I tried when we were first married to get enthusiastic about sex. It never felt right. I loved Roger. I just wanted to be normal. I hoped it would get better but it hasn't. He is more outgoing than me. He joined the local amateur theatre group recently. That's where he met her. I know he wanted more sex and I'm not keen. I don't blame him. He takes great care of me. He says the affair is over but I'm frightened he'll leave me."

She rocked herself back and forward.

I wondered how they dealt with other problems but I preferred to talk to them together.

Reluctantly Elaine agreed to return with Roger.

At the second consultation, Elaine sat on the edge of the chair. Her right foot flicked up and down endlessly. Her gaze was glued to a fixed spot on the floor. She never raised her eyes in contact. Roger was also uncomfortable.

"I feel such a fool having the affair. I love Elaine but since the kids left, the house has felt empty."

It is easy to assume that an affair can start because sex is not good at home, but that is only skimming the surface. The reasons generally go deeper. An affair is a common distraction when a couple is in troubled waters. It may be tempting to leave the marriage partner because you feel wonderful with your new love. But it is unlikely that you have found someone who suits you better, usually you have found someone who simply knows less about you.

The one who finds another love has found a way to sidestep the differences that emerge in marriage. The classic line, 'My wife (husband) doesn't understand me,' is far from the truth. She (he) understands a great deal and says what she (he) does not like. She would like him to change. He would like her to change. It can be hard to face these challenges.

It may seem easier to find a lover and enjoy the oblivion of the mists of honeymoon. As an added bonus sex can be intensely exciting given little knowledge of each other, no reality and the spice of clandestine encounters. Roger had tried an affair but it had not provided any lasting solution. He needed to address his feeling of being empty inside which he had phrased as the house being empty.

Neither Elaine nor Roger knew what else to do. I find couples have generally tried very hard to resolve differences before seeking counselling. It was important they acknowledged their efforts to date so as not to sink into despair. I asked what they had done so far when problems arose.

"I'd try to talk to Elaine. But she'd get upset and cry or walk away. Then she wouldn't speak to me for days even when I pleaded with her. I'd just feel bad and give up. Now we talk about day-to-day things, the kids problems but not our own."

Elaine was silent so I asked her directly if that was a fair view.

"Yes, but I get hurt when he criticises me. I can't bear to argue. I just

want peace. I think it's better to walk away than say something you might regret. Things always settle down."

Her foot stilled as she spoke this last sentence.

They certainly settled down but nothing personal was ever resolved. I wonder how Roger coped when Elaine walked away.

"It's OK really. I don't like it when Elaine goes quiet on me but I agree that it's better than an argument. I used to try to get her to talk but I gave up. It's a waste of time."

They had developed a tolerable style of dealing with a problem. They avoided open conflict like the plague. But what became hidden in the depths and at what cost?

Compare this list of questions on 'hidden conflict' to that on page 136 concerning 'open conflict' and you will see they are very similar.

In hidden conflict

Have you:
- silently blamed the other?
- had a fixed mind?
- tried to please the other by sacrificing your own desires?
- been stressed?
- expected your partner to relieve that stress?
- found distractions to avoid dealing with a problem, e.g., TV, excessive work?
- not been open to accepting your partner's view as right for them?
- expected a partner to read your mind?
- had an expectation of how your partner should be?
- not acknowledged your own concerns, but projected them as coming from your partner?
- translated one occasion to always?
- swallowed your anger?

- not shared how you felt?
- walked away?
- avoided talking about the problem again?

Open and hidden conflict appear entirely different on the surface. In fact both are win/lose conflict techniques. Open conflict is more obvious. The more subtle response of withdrawal from a problem still creates distance from each other. Hidden or open, conflict leads to resentment and pain. Greg and Pauline, Elaine and Roger had experienced similar sexual outcomes of low sexual interest in one partner. It is not surprising when you realise both couples tried to go around their problems rather than through them.

Win/lose attempts to discuss differences leave you stuck. You feel trapped in a vicious cycle. Round and round you go. Nothing changes except that the level of resentment escalates. There are no winners in the long term. There are better ways to discuss difference that release you from inertia. Before 'charting new waters' it is worth understanding why you have been going round in circles.

Of the so called 'resolutions' (page 136) in win/lose conflict most clearly get you nowhere. The one you may accept too readily is 'compromise'. You may wonder what could be wrong with compromise as a solution to conflict. It is held up as the essential ingredient to hold a relationship together. But you can sacrifice your self and intimacy as a result of compromise. If you make a deal that leaves you with a heavy heart, what does this do to your desire for life and for each other?

Unhealthy compromise

Let us return for a final glimpse at the way Marianne and Joe had run into trouble. They had compromised on their holiday destination (and many other issues in their relationship). Marianne wanted to go on holiday to the mountains to ski. Joe wanted to go on holiday to the beach to surf. They also wanted to take a holiday together. They compromised and agreed to go surfing this year and skiing next year.

On the surface this seems good. But Marianne accompanied Joe on the beach holiday full of resentment. She complained about the heat, the sand and the terrible accommodation. They had created the recipe for a lousy holiday (and lousy sex).

Outwardly Marianne appeared to compromise but in her heart she was resentful at not getting what she wanted. If the following year they had gone skiing and Joe injured his knee you can imagine whom he would blame.

Unhealthy compromise, to please the other, leads to resentment, which usually gets acted out. In the end the other 'pays' for 'making' you do what you did not want to do.

There is an alternative to compromise in the form of a healthy adjustment. In this you can explore both viewpoints with an open mind.

When you have fully considered all possibilities you may find your final choice is not the one you originally planned. You have made a healthy adjustment that feels completely right to you. This is discussed in further depth in the next section, Charting New Waters.

Jane and Robert had made healthy adjustment in several areas of their life but you might recall their approach to sex was accepting what they thought could not be changed though sex was not fulfilling for either. Eventually they sought therapy to gain a fresh perspective.

Jane and Robert had liked most of what they saw in each other. They gradually began to reveal more of their likes and dislikes to each other. Their love was maturing beyond Provisional Love. But there was one particular area that was still limiting this maturation –sexuality.

Jane settled comfortably into the chair.

"We spent a lot of time together in the first 18 months getting to

know each other. Then we decided to get engaged. We moved in together. It took some time to get used to each other's ways. Robert wanted me to cook dinner each night. I hate cooking and I hadn't told him before. But he was great when I did. We decided to share that chore and it works OK. We have some laughs in the kitchen. We eat some takeaway too."

Jane had finally told Robert of her disinterest in cooking. She did not want to pretend she liked cooking but they did need to eat. Therefore they reached a healthy adjustment. They shared the responsibility and made it fun.

"She was untidy and I like things neat. My Mum had always kept the house super tidy. In some ways it was good that with Jane I could relax a bit more. It was a challenge at first but I found I could cope with some things lying around. It seems more balanced.

"There was a really comfortable feeling between us so we planned our wedding. Even with this sex thing I'm still glad we did."

They had entered marriage for many positive reasons. They were able to discuss several differences. Robert had reviewed his idea that the house should be tidy. He could be relaxed about less time directed to housework. It freed time for other activities. He opened his mind to understand Jane's way and chose to make an adjustment to his old thinking. He had not compromised his belief on tidiness. He had reconsidered his view taking into account his new circumstance. He decided he could benefit from a change of thinking. But in sex they had compromised.

"The sex problem has been the hardest to talk about. I would like us to have a better sex life. It isn't normal not to be able to do it properly. But when we talk about it, I get upset. We've settled on sex without penetration. We've managed that for six years but it isn't right. We pretended it was OK but I worry that Robert will get fed up and leave."

"No I want this marriage to work. Whatever it takes I will give it a go. I don't want to push Jane but I would like a normal sex life.'

"So would I," Jane whispered.

Jane and Robert were navigating troubled waters. They had maintained goodwill but even so could not come close to dealing with the sex problem; their compromise left each with a heavy heart. They had a sex life that fell short of what they wanted. By not talking about sex they could avoid most of their distress. They had tolerated being sexual but never having penetration. They both reached orgasm but finally, tolerable was not enough. They had avoided their concerns on unfulfilled sexuality by making this a taboo topic. If they had not started to talk about having children they might have been able to continue with these avoidance techniques for even longer.

It was going to take delving into the depths of their beliefs to find reasons for this problem and then establish ways to make change. It would take revealing more than they had ever done before. It meant facing some of their limiting fears. Not settling for a compromise, not avoiding the problem, but finally facing up to their problem.

Sex in troubled waters

Whether you fight over who steered the love boat into trouble or try to ignore the storms, you will still be uncomfortably buffeted around when you seek comfort in the bedroom. You may be able to hide distress in all other areas of your relationship but sex in troubled waters will in some way reveal your differences.

Desire differences, erectile problems, orgasm difficulties or unusual sexual behaviour, you name it, there is always an interaction of the physical and emotional to be considered. It is a normal human response for sexuality to be reflective of the state of the relationship and other personal issues.

It is tempting to blame someone or something for a problem with sex. It would be easier if a single reason with a simple solution could be found but rarely is this true. Check through this list, would you ever use one of these to explain away a sex problem to your self?

Simple reasons for sex problems

- I/my partner doesn't know enough about sex.
- It's the contraceptive we use.
- I/my partner isn't a good lover.
- My sexy bits are the wrong shape or size.
- I have a low sex drive.
- I don't have an orgasm.
- I come too quickly.
- My erection isn't so good any more.
- I have had a baby.
- It's because of menopause.
- It's my age.
- I was abused.
- I am disabled.
- Maybe I'm gay/lesbian.

If you use one of these reasons to explain a problem you may find the love boat stuck on a sandbank. These are not solutions and can become excuses allowing you to accept rather than consider change in the situation.

These reasons need to be placed in the context of your whole life. You need to include all of the factors that were discussed in Part One of the book that contribute to who you are and any problems you encounter.

To recap they include:
- childhood learning

- culture
- gender
- health
- your beliefs

and in addition:

- the stage and state of your relationship
- who you are deep inside

It is important not to jump at the simple single reason for a problem. It is wise to honour your complexity as a human being. Elaine and Roger, Marianne and Joe, Greg and Pauline certainly had a multitude of reasons for their sexual problems. They are real people with real differences between them and the real dilemma of how to cope with being together.

I am even more concerned when a couple say that for some inexplicable reason they have no differences between them – except in sex. They are often unknowingly disguising their differences. Scared that the only alternative to revealing difference is to leave (or even worse to be left) a cover-up of problems seems preferable.

You may think of low desire as some kind of illness, but what could be more natural when your feelings are confused. During troubled times it is normal for desire to alter. As differences become known, although not resolved, it is often that one partner becomes less interested in sex as a sign of their resentment while the other partner then pursues sex. Each is expressing, in the bedroom, their disappointment with problems that exist outside the bedroom. The source of a problem needs to be addressed when and where it occurs, not held over to be acted out sexually.

If you feel that your partner controls your life outside the bedroom, you may be the one who says, 'No'. You gain control of sex, if nothing else. This rarely occurs at a conscious level but at a subtler one in the unconscious mind. Thus, sex, often unknowingly, gets drawn into win/lose conflict.

Early in a relationship both may enjoy sex, your feelings reinforced by your similarities and out of desire to please each other. But you do not know each other well in the early stage of a relationship. You know what you agree upon but much disagreement still lies hidden.

It is easy to reveal sexual and inner feelings that you know meet the approval of the other. This is the realm of Provisional Love. However, when the stage of the relationship is reached when differences begin to emerge and often are met with disapproval it is less easy to reveal who you are and what you want. This has a flow-on effect to sex.

In the two couples – Pauline and Greg, Elaine and Roger, it was the woman who showed a lower sexual desire. Both women, however, did desire a pleasurable sex life. Contrary to popular belief low desire for sex occurs in men as well as women. In my own practice men accounted for approximately 25% of those who presented with low desire. The higher frequency of women revealing they are in trouble waters by having low interest in sex may result from the way men and women display intimacy.

As discussed in the chapter on the effects of gender roles (Boy Meets Girl), for some people (particularly men) the way they learn to be intimate is to have sex with their beloved. Wishing to recapture the intimacy, which seems lost during difficult times, sexual intercourse is often pursued. Talking from their heart is a harder way to maintain intimacy.

Some people (particularly women) experience intimacy through sharing inner thoughts and feelings with another. Females do this throughout life with girlfriends and later their sexual partner. It makes sense to a woman to pursue verbal intercourse to re-establish intimacy. When this route fails there is little desire to share sex when there appears to be no intimacy. Each considers the route with which he/she is comfortable to be the right and normal way. Neither is wrong. Both are seeking the same thing - to be close to their partner. To be able to include both physical and emotional connection is respectful of both.

Beyond troubled waters

I was once asked during a workshop, "Why don't people sort all this stuff out before they make a commitment?" This is a good question but it raises many more. Taking time before commitment helps reveal some important differences. But how much time do you take to reveal who you really are? Do you want to? Do you know who you are? Do you commit to a relationship at the cost of your self? Do you have the courage to commit to being your self? Or is the whole purpose of sharing the love boat to find answers to these questions?

Can you come to know your self and reveal who you are through love and sex? Or does the thought of revealing your self make you feel vulnerable, at risk of being hurt? You may get 'loved' by hiding much of your self from another and this deception may provide you with a partner - but not a lasting happiness. Even if you are married you do not own anyone.

When the unhappiness of not being your self in a relationship finally surfaces you face a challenge. Will you abandon ship to set sail with someone else, or explore the freedom of being open and honest and risk being loved for who you are? This opportunity often arises in troubled waters. You may fail to seize it if your only aim is to survive the storm.

But you can go beyond surviving to thriving.

You can question your own beliefs, extend your abilities in understanding differences and most of all learn to be true to your self. This offers the excitement and fear of setting your own course perhaps for the first time in your life. If a beloved can do the same you may find yourselves discovering that you truly desire to be together at that moment.

The love boat always sails into troubled waters and will challenge you.

As you take the helm and navigate through the storm with a view to a new course you need your eyes, your heart and your mind open. You will both experience change and may, for a while, be unsure if you wish to continue your voyage together. Be willing to 'chart new waters'. Expanding how you relate can steer you away from win/lose conflict into respectful discussion of problems. You will come to know your self better and come to know your partner better.

Before you plan your new course it helps to understand how and why you headed into troubled waters, an area which was not marked on any chart when you set sail. Elaine and Roger, Jane and Robert, Greg and Pauline discovered this offered them new possibilities for their future voyage.

*You don't bring me flowers.
You don't sing me love songs.
You hardly talk to me anymore
When you come through the door at the end of the day.*

'You don't bring me flowers'
Neil Diamond

Chapter Eleven

The voyage becomes a challenge

Starting 'in love' everything seems possible. As you embark on the love boat 'happily ever after' feels automatic. There is a wonderful combination of Agape and Eros to accompany you on your cruise. Why do you now find your self challenged by storms on your voyage? Why does a relationship 'go wrong'? Why does it seem hard to enjoy continuing love and sex? You can examine some of the common reasons that problems arise:

Incompatibility

Clearly, some people choose the wrong partner. They rush into a commitment to the relationship rather than taking time to get to know each other. Like Marianne and Joe, they are incompatible. But others have good reasons to be together and the bond of their love is strong. Still they enter troubled waters. They experience the distress of conflict, whether this is out in the open or suppressed in withdrawal. There are a variety of factors which contribute to the gathering storms:

The pressures of life

Much as you might hope to ignore the many pressures associated with modern lifestyle and relationships you find you cannot. In response to the stress created you find your self reacting automatically rather than taking time to think. You feel a tight knot in your stomach or throat, sweating, racing pulse, or being irritable. Stress is unpleasant for you and your partner. Learning to relax, however, may be easier said than done. Stress management techniques are useful but you may not have the time to meditate, do yoga or take a walk. Do you even allow your self the time to take a deep breath? Try taking one now and ask your self if your life has become an endless performance, with no time to relax. If you personally are in this state, what effect does this have on your relationship?

'In love' you took the time to do things that brought delight. Picnics, walks, a funny movie, dinner out, sharing an interest, laying in bed together on a Sunday morning sprinkled your life with stardust. Life easily becomes so busy and complex that you no longer have time to do anything that gives you pleasure. In a life devoid of enjoyment, you may squeeze sex into a spare 10 minutes and expect intercourse to be so fantastic as to substitute for all the diverse activities you used to enjoy. This particular expectation needs a reality check!

You need quality time for your self and together for any chance of happiness in love and sex. Do you remember how you talked for hours when you were in love? Not just chatter, but life, the universe and everything. Have you run out of things to talk about or is it the way that you talk to each other that has changed?

Greg and Pauline, Elaine and Roger struggled in win/lose conflict and no longer enjoyed talking to each other. They found distractions they called pressures of life to keep them apart. But which is the chicken and which the egg? They needed to review the reasons for their busyness and find a better way to communicate.

Difference

Perhaps you talk less because you are no longer in the comfort zone of similarity. In the limited time you allow for talking, do you find your self complaining about your differences and problems? Although no two people are alike, our culture does not encourage you to honour difference. Black and white, man and woman, old and young, rich and poor, hetero or homosexual we do not understand each other easily. You would like others to be the same as you, not different. 'In love' you celebrate the similarity of your self and your partner. Later you may think you are opposites.

What makes each one unique? Some personality traits may be inherited but science does not know which are and which are not. Genes however are influenced by the environment in which you grew up. Many behaviour patterns develop in response to your family members. Since your partner's family may be as different as chalk from cheese to yours, you will need some skills to respect differences between you. This is a challenge if you have not learned these skills when you were growing up. But it is never too late to learn and respectful discussion is explained in detail in Chapter Twelve.

Fixed roles

You may have fallen into defined roles in your relationship. These may have suited you early on, but are no longer appropriate. A relationship can 'go wrong' because of the inflexibility of established roles. When you were growing up you tested limits all the time. As you continue to mature you still want to extend your limits. You started the voyage in the honeymoon suite and now you are chopping vegetables down in the galley! Do you plan a spectacular escape or will you allow your self to breathe some fresh air on deck?

Behaviour patterns

Early in the relationship you may not reveal your usual behaviours. You want to impress, you buy new clothes, turn up on time, even cancel a meeting to share champagne in bed. Later, old behaviours stubbornly return. Behaviour does not change long term, unless there is also a change in underlying thinking.

Here are a few typical examples of old behaviour that may re-emerge in your partner:

	In love	**In troubled waters**
You go out for the evening.	He/she dresses to impress.	He/she is scruffy.
He/she is stressed.	He/she has a drink.	He/she gets drunk.
You have an idea.	He/she listens.	He/she criticises.

You can make your own list of the ways your partner behaves that are different from when you met. You will probably find it much harder to make the same list about your self. These examples will help you to begin:

	In love	**In troubled waters**
He/she disagrees with you.	You smile and listen.	You get angry.
You want sex he/she doesn't.	You say, "that's fine,"	You act coldly.
You hate your job.	You tell.	You don't tell.

In addition is the behaviour you 'accepted' earlier but never liked. Perhaps you hoped that eventually he/she would change of their own accord. It is a rude awakening to realise that this has not happened and probably will not. You might stop trying to make the other change and bear resentment instead. Alternatively, you may intensify your efforts to make your partner become what you want. Often the harder you push the more they resist.

While you are trying to change your partner he/she is just as intent on changing you. As a child you learned to adapt your self, often to suit your parents. Now your partner wants you to alter again. It is no wonder you feel uncomfortable. When do you get to be your self?

Many of your responses were learned as a child. Some have remained unrefined since then. Some your beloved does not like. Some you do not like. Many have been absorbed from others rather than being right for your self. Some would benefit from being modified. To do this is a challenge of your voyage.

Self esteem

In troubled waters self esteem is rarely high. You may have lost (or never found) confidence in who you are. It can be particularly confusing to find you are assured in one part of life such as work but not in your personal life.

Elaine expressed from where she hoped to obtain esteem:

"If only Roger paid me more attention and didn't criticise so much, I'd have self esteem."

In these words Elaine revealed a common misconception about self esteem. No one else can give you self esteem that must come from within.

While the 'in love' phase is littered with compliments, you can be sure that in troubled waters there will be few. Your esteem can plummet if it has been dependent on the goodwill of your partner. You can hope or beg for more positive remarks from your partner but he/she can no longer supply your needs. If you become focused on the dream that someone new will make you feel good, your relationship deteriorates further. If you focus on renewing your self, you gain a fresh view that may revitalise your relationship.

Unfortunately, the deal made early in your relationship, to receive a positive boost to your esteem, may have been to give up any aspects of your self that might rock the boat. Eventually when you cannot suppress your self any longer you may stand up shouting, 'What about me?' The love boat sways precariously but now you cannot simply sit down quietly. Change has become inevitable.

Disappointment in love and sex

When you feel disillusioned and disappointed with love or sex you find defenses learned in the past are quickly activated rather than thinking through a situation. Jealousy, fear of loss, anger, frustration, withdrawal are common when you are struggling in troubled waters to keep your relationship afloat. These emotions are at odds with love. Each contribute to a relationship 'going wrong'. We saw how they affect a relationship in the last two chapters. It is worthwhile to revisit the reasons for distress in a relationship to understand why .

As you follow Greg and Pauline, Elaine and Roger you will understand why they are facing a stormy passage. However, their relationships are not going wrong. In fact, the challenges of the voyage are steering them towards mature love.

The pressures of life

Greg wanted to talk about stresses that affected him.

"Pauline doesn't work. We both wanted her to care for the children. I wanted her to be proud of me. My parents taught me, to get ahead you have to work hard. I started a furniture business. Now there is so much competition from bigger companies who can import cheaply. I have to keep my prices down. I worry about paying bills and staff. I borrowed to buy the factory but the repayments are high. It's a good investment for the future but it's touch and go some months. I work longer hours than ever to earn the same amount. I don't get home until late most nights. I take my responsibilities seriously."

I wondered if it had always been this way. Was Greg's life always so burdened?

"*Well, before the kids I was busy setting up a new business. It was hard work but it was exciting. But I seemed to get through more in less time. I looked forward to getting home to Pauline.*" A smile slipped onto his face.

This sounded like a common problem. When 'in love' Greg had energy for work and found time to be with Pauline. Then came a shift in focus. He returned to the weighty duty of being financially successful.

There are many pressures in modern life, particularly financial ones, but there are choices about how to live. Greg's parents had placed much emphasis on the rewards that hard work and money were expected to bring - security and love. But for Greg both love and security were in doubt.

Were the standards set by Greg's parents right for what he wanted now? Had Greg ever stopped to consider what he really wanted for himself?

Concern about money can mask underlying concerns for happiness, security, most of all love. Was it pressure of work that meant Greg came home late or had work become a distraction from problems?

Modern life is extremely busy. Everyone has so much to do that it is easy to forget to be. It need not be this way. It requires effort to challenge expectations learned early on life but you can reset the balance. In an early relationship much time is dedicated to being together. When work, financial considerations and children become part of the relationship it can be difficult to remember to have quality time together.

Time together is desired only when it feels good. The 'Catch 22' is that it takes time to sort things out so that you can feel good. You have to be willing to spend time talking and working through the difficulties. There are no short cuts.

Fixed roles

Pauline and Greg had adopted fixed roles in their marriage. Greg was the provider of money. Pauline was home carer and mother. This suited them at first but now neither were finding these roles entirely to their liking. Pauline wanted to review the original deal of their marriage. This inevitably heralded change.

"He's right we did agree that I stay home and raise the children. But now I'm fed up with that. I want to do more. That's why I started to study. I don't want to be home all the time when Greg comes home. I want a life. I want to be more than a mother and wife." Pauline was very definite.

You enter a relationship with a foundation of family and social rules. You may slip into a role in response to these influences, often unaware of this at a conscious level. The traditional deal is for each to be the provider of certain services. But does this deal involve unhealthy compromise? Does it allow for change?

Inflexible roles have the apparent security of knowing what to expect. This is, in fact, the last thing you get from Provisional Love. You have not revealed your all, so you are bound to be in for a few surprises. Can you grow with the unexpected?

Greg was finding this very difficult.

"I don't know why she isn't satisfied. I've done everything for her. I get so angry when she talks like this."

Greg was back trying to control the relationship. Using anger he was trying to prevent change. He was struggling with his fear of the unknown. But Greg and Pauline could both benefit from reviewing their roles. Both were fed up with the responsibility for the other and not for themselves. Change had something to offer. Being stationary can seem safe but the real safety lies in being able to adapt.

In their roles, Pauline prepared the meals, cared for the children, did the household chores. Pauline identified herself as a good mother and wife. Greg worked hard and made money. He described himself as a good father and provider. Caught in treating each other as though their roles were all they were, there was little chance for mature intimacy to flourish. Their relationship was dependent on fulfilling predictable roles. Where was love? Where was desire?

Once again it is in sexuality that the limitation of roles is reflected. Mentally limited to performing as a wife and mother, the last thing Pauline felt like was sex. Feeling sexy is about how you feel inside and cannot be prescribed by an external role. But she did feel guilty because Greg needed sex. She felt duty bound to provide it. Greg in his role took the responsibility to make things happen, including sex. Over the years the provision of sex rather than the desire for it had become the norm.

To open your self to follow your heart, first you need to know what your true desires are. If roles and old patterns of behaviour feel like limits, they probably are. You may not be used to listening to your own intuition but it is a reliable guidance. You decide what feels right to continue and what feels better to change. To do this you need to identify what has been unthinkingly absorbed from others in the past and reassess its value in your present. Your own wisdom, not that of your parents, friends, partner or society is your guide.

Patterns of thought and behaviour

Many patterns of behaviour begin in childhood in attempts to gain love or attention from your mother and father. You are enjoying just being your self when you hear the disapproving voice, "Don't do that, it's naughty/ bad/ wrong." To regain approval you learn to alter your self. Gradually you are shaped, patterned, moulded by others so that your original self becomes restrained. You present an image to the world modified to suit other people.

Parents generally strive to use their authority to pass their standards on to children. As you grow you learn to develop your own standards. Eventually you do not need to check with anyone else what you choose to think or do. But surprisingly often you do just that. Parental values often remain in your memory long after they are appropriate to your own life.

Part of maturing is to review your lessons – discard some, update some and hold on to what suits your present circumstances.

Some learning made sense to your childhood but is now outdated. Habit keeps you accessing it long past its 'use by' date. I can recall an example from my own life.

"*I came from a family in which money was limited. Every purchase had to be seriously considered and serve a multitude of purposes. I have a love of colour. It is an integral part of me that brings me much joy. As a child it wasn't always possible to enjoy my colour passion as often as I wanted to. Black was sensible. This learning had advantages later when I was an impoverished student. I knew how to make a sensible purchase and spend less money. Later in life I had a comfortable income. But I still acted in the old way.*

"*I was in Hong Kong. My eyes were feasting on a pair of turquoise suede shoes trimmed with snakeskin, in a shop window. I knew I wanted them. I tried on the shoes. They were perfect. The helpful shop assistant showed me the same shoes – in black. I hesitated, black would go with more things, not get so dirty. My heart said the turquoise, my head said the black. I dithered for 10 minutes... and bought the black pair.*

"*My husband (now ex) had come from a family that was more comfortable financially than mine. He was perplexed by my decision. For him my dilemma made no sense. His learning had been if you want something, you buy it.*

"*Outside the shop I once more gazed at the turquoise pair in the window. The black pair (my compromise) dangled heavily on my arm in the shopping bag. He saw the look on my face and told me to buy the turquoise ones. Back into the shop I went, this time I took the ones I wanted. Those shoes brought me so much delight I wore them till they fell to bits.*"

I had learned to be careful when spending money. It was the only option as a child. In doing so I had to subdue my desire for colour. I had buried a small part of myself in the process. Even when I earned my own living and it was reasonable to express this buried desire, I could not allow myself to. I was stuck with learning that was ingrained. Part of me thought it was wrong to indulge in an impractical purchase. It took some encouragement from my husband for me to break that habit. He could do it easily because he always had. He had learned a different way in his family.

This is a light-hearted look at updating a way of thinking in line with changed adult circumstances. But it carries important messages. It shows how a partner can be mystified by your limits when they had a different learning experience. This difference is confronting and you are presented with another view to consider. You balance your old thinking with this new option, giving you the chance to break a habit. You use whichever seems most appropriate in a particular circumstance. Any change that occurs is decided by you. It is not up to your partner to tell you what to do but he/she does help you confront your learned patterns. If the challenge slips into 'I'm right, you're wrong', you are thrown in the win/lose conflict of troubled waters.

How do you learn things in the first place? You receive information through your senses – hearing, sight, taste, smell, touch. You have an emotional response and thinking is stimulated.

You pick up a lemon for the first time. It is a pretty colour. It smells good. You bite into it. Ugh! it tastes terrible. You feel terrible. You think, 'I'll never eat one of those again.' All this is stored in your memory and you learn. You adopt the belief that lemons are horrible. Does that memory limit you? How do you learn to make lemon meringue pie unless you are willing to update this memory?

Some events are more disturbing and lead to painful memories. It may be a series of minor upsets or a single trauma that is stored as an unhappy memory. You are the only judge of what troubled you as a child. In this we are very individual. If you have suffered emotional, physical or sexual abuse, your world as a child was distorted by the dysfunction of the abuser. This learning may restrict the ease of your function later in life. If you feel limited by your early experiences, counselling can be invaluable in sorting through the remaining pain and in assisting you to choose a way to live now that reopens your heart to enjoy the present.

Even as a child you find a way to cope with a turmoil of feelings. You may hide them deep in your mind. You hope you will never have to suffer such a bad feeling ever again. The stored memory contributes to what you believe. The problem with a buried feeling and the belief it generates is that both stay deprived of growth and change. Someone says or does something that triggers the old bad feeling and you have your emotions churned up in a flash.

You can try pushing them down deeper or take the opportunity to shed some light on the incomplete knowledge.

New Age literature uses words such as 'child within', 'inner child' or 'wounded child' to consider the child-learned thinking, beliefs and behaviours that limit you. But these are diminutive words. You are an adult and know you have gone beyond childish things. You have put away your toys, taken the responsibility for finances, perhaps married, raised children – these are clearly adult behaviours. You need to utilise your adult strengths to update the remnants of child-learned behaviour that limit your maturity.

A shift to an inner focus does allow you to identify the origin of your limitations. At first you may righteously experience angry outbursts as you blame parents or others for your present difficulties in life. Growth requires more. It is important to acknowledge the source of distress in childhood and mature your responses. This is the substance of growing up.

Some learning results from feeling that a need, whether reasonable or unreasonable, was not met by a parent or other loved one. As a child you try to get these needs met appropriately using childlike behaviour such as sulking, crying or yelling. Expecting someone else to meet your needs is a leftover from childhood. The behaviour you use now to achieve this end may still date from this period. These expectations limit your independence. An update is required if you want to be fulfilled in the present rather than be limited by your past.

Perhaps the deepest need that a human being knows is the need to experience love. It is this area that requires most awareness, insight and effort to mature. Love is a classic unmet need, one you may expect someone else to fulfil. Romantic tales support this expectation. The knight in shining armour will take care of you. The damsel will make you feel like a king. 'In love' fulfils your need for a while, troubled waters do not. The disappointment of this reality can present the opportunity to discover how to love yourself. New understanding will often emerge during times of crisis. The storm often stimulates the remnant of a childish need to surface and be expressed. It is hard to break the pattern of neediness in love and sex. But continuation of this neediness is a major cause of unhappiness.

In Chapter Eight Peter (page 118) was needy for attention. His wife Judy had fulfilled his need until they had a baby which demanded much of her time. Peter found someone else to give him attention and had an affair. When Judy found out she told him she wanted to leave him. Peter was awakened to the devastation that his neediness could bring.

"I felt neglected when the baby came along. Then Judy wasn't interested in sex. I felt she didn't care about me anymore. Just like I did when I was growing up. There were seven of us. I never remember Mum having time for me. She was always fussing over one of the little ones."

In therapy he talked about how emotionally neglected he felt because his mother placed her attention on the younger children. The more he talked the more he shifted from a child's perspective of 'give me' to add his adult awareness of how it must have been to bring up seven children. He was struggling with only one. He no longer felt deprived and rather then resent his son he opened his heart to him and found he could share his love with his wife, his son and himself. Judy had needed to mother Peter and she had shifted her need to mother onto the baby. She also grew beyond her need and learned to value herself as well as the baby and Peter.

In both love and sex you may expect that someone will take care of you. There is more lightness in your heart and theirs when someone cares about you. You have the freedom to care for someone when you have learned to care for your self.

Your behaviour and thoughts are not fixed. They are open to change though change will take effort. Listen to your own inner voice. If you continue to be directed by the external voice of another, as you were when a child, you will struggle.

Models for learning

If you had perfect parents you would have learned all about respect and equality from them. You would be skilled at listening to your own

intuition. Your perfect parents would have:
- been role models of equality and intimacy
- worked on their own selves and marriage and reached mature love
- had done most of this before kids came on the scene and distracted them totally
- shared their wisdom with you

It is more likely that your parents were mere mortals with heaps of unresolved issues and limited energy to sort them out. They just did the best they could. Few families demonstrate the skills required to sort out differences in a compassionate way.

Good models of balanced mature loving are rare. We tend to have models of open or suppressed anger and struggle. At home, at school and through the media you are swamped with win/lose examples. From the fantasy of television 'soapies' through to real life war, relationships are portrayed as opportunities to win or lose.

Self esteem

To move beyond the limits of childhood you require self esteem. This is the regard for your self that you gain by self care. No one else can provide you with self esteem. You start out life full of joy with a self will that can direct you in life. If you are heavily influenced by others, you forget to listen to your own heart, and lose contact with delight. You may find your self joyless by the time your relationship is in troubled waters.

Self esteem can be slowly eroded by the 'give and take' that you are told to value. When you do something that you do not want to and you feel a heaviness in your heart, you have made an unhealthy compromise. When you please someone else but harbour resentment, you give up a part of your joy. But is is possible to build self esteem and regain joy, once you come to understand your own process of loss of esteem.

Elaine was struggling to understand herself. She began by reviewing her past.

"My Mum had always been there for us and for Dad. She was up early each morning to prepare breakfast. She packed our lunches. Mum took so much time making special treats for dinner. The house was always clean. She was such a lovely person. She had time for everyone. She used to help out the nuns clean the church. Dad wasn't home much.

"I remember Mum was often sad. She used to say, 'I don't know what I'd do without you, Elaine.' I tried so hard to please her, to cheer her up."

Elaine thought she had a perfect mother, unselfish and giving. She took responsibility to reduce her mother's sadness by doing her best to please.

"There was a terrible time when I was 13. I was at Convent School. The nuns called Mum in, said I was spending too much time with an older girl, my friend Jenny. 'It won't do,' they said. 'It isn't natural.' Mum was devastated. 'How could you behave like that after all I've done for you. I'll never live down the embarrassment,' she said. Then she hardly spoke to me for weeks. I didn't understand. I just knew that somehow they all thought my having a girlfriend was wrong. So I stopped talking to Jenny."

Elaine's mother had set the scene. She did take care of every one else. But she never let them forget her self sacrifice. She was clearly unhappy. Elaine recognised the sacrifices her mother made and felt she should do the same in return. She learned as a child that to gain her mother's love she must please her.

Her occasional attempts to be self directing were met with disapproval. She felt the silent punishment of withdrawal of love. As Elaine talked more she recalled this withdrawal had happened many times in her childhood.

"You know, I think the nuns were cruel to treat me that way. I really needed Mum to explain but she was so cold. I wanted to be loved. If ever I did anything wrong, Mum would tell me off then she'd sit down and cry. I'd try hard to be good to make her feel better."

Elaine directed her focus on making her mother feel better. She was desperate to regain her love. Deep in the hiding place in her mind Elaine had buried the fear 'I am not lovable unless I do what someone else expects'. To be loved Elaine had to sacrifice her own desires. She lost herself in her growing years. Marriage continued the process.

"I wasn't interested in boys, until I met Roger. He was very kind. Mum was so delighted when we got engaged. I wanted to get married and have children. I wanted to be like everyone else.

"Roger loves me. I try to do everything to please him in return. But I just can't do sex anymore. I feel so hopeless."

In these words Elaine made clear the trade she made. She placed her focus on pleasing Roger in return for his love. She had learned this as a child.

I asked how Roger behaved when he did not like something she had done.

"He tells me what I've done wrong in his teacher's voice. I feel so bad I don't know what to say. Then he is very distant for a while. But I know how to fix things, I cook his favourite dinner and he comes around."

In this situation, Roger behaved in the same way as Elaine's mother. In response, Elaine behaved as she had as a child. She paid little attention to her own wants. To gain love she tried to please Roger rather than be herself, just as she had with her mother.

"But I know Mum loved me. Look at all she did."

I wondered if Elaine had thought what she meant by 'love'. I gave her the definitions of love (Chapter Six) to take away and think about.

She returned with the questionnaire filled in for all the family members and friends.

"That really made me think. I sat and stared at the questionnaire. I was anxious about filling it out. In the end I did. I'd like to show you."

She passed over the paper, unable to put her feelings into words. Elaine had assessed the love she felt for mother as Philia, Provisional and Dependent. She thought her mother loved her in the same ways. Her assessment of her feelings for Roger were Philia and Provisional.

"Neither of them know me. How can they when I hardly know myself. That's why I put provisional love."

She knew she wanted more. Nowhere in the chart had Elaine ticked Eros. I wondered if she had ever felt this. I asked her.

Elaine blushed and started to wring her hands. "I... er, did with Jenny – Eros and Agape. She accepted me just as I am. It was a wonderful feeling. I've never forgotten. But it has worried me my whole life. Oh God! Do you think I'm a lesbian?"

This was the first time she had voiced her possible desire and fear. It would have been simple for me to answer 'yes' and pat myself on the back for getting to the bottom of Elaine's problem. Instead, I respected that Elaine needed time to answer this for herself. Labelling Elaine as lesbian would have been a simplistic explanation of all her problems. Is sexual desire exclusively hetero or homosexual in nature or can it be stirred by sharing love (Agape) with another, independent of gender? In love may Agape flow onto Eros? Is the choice of the gender of a partner part of an independent discovery of your self?

In all honesty, Elaine had been out of touch with her own desires for most of her life. She could not answer the question of gender preference yet. There was no escaping the work Elaine had to do to regain her self awareness. She could begin by exploring her sexual feelings and other buried discomforts. Brought to the surface she could use her adult knowledge to challenge the beliefs which had been trapped in a time warp and not matured. Elaine had lost herself in this marriage. Roger had done the same. He spoke on his own, about his affair.

"Elaine is kind. Yet it's hard for me to say what I want, if it's different from her. Most of the time I try to fit in. But sometimes I want to be myself. For years I wanted to join the local drama society. I love the theatre. Elaine asked me not to. She said she'd be lonely in the evening. She'd well up in tears. Then if I tried to talk she'd say I lecture her. I'd stay home with her and watch TV. It didn't seem a lot to give up. But this year I felt so restricted that I finally went along. That feeling of not being able to do what I want made me feel trapped. That's one of the reasons I had the affair."

Roger gave up the part of himself that loved theatre – to please Elaine, to keep the relationship. Have you done this to maintain your relationship? You may think part of commitment is to go along with each other. But is your commitment to the relationship at the price of your self? There is a point in life when you want to be your self, when it would feel good to be loved for your self, not for the sacrifices you make.

"I wanted to talk to Elaine about my leaving teaching but she wouldn't listen. She kept asking what would we do for money."

Roger wanted to make a change. He had finally admitted to himself that he did not like his job. He wanted to explore other possibilities. He wanted to share this dilemma with Elaine. Fearful of change she wanted him to continue his job. She did not try to understand the review he wanted of his professional life. She wanted to keep him on the straight and narrow.

The desire to recommence education, take a job, change a job, take a new interest is often the real 'you' emerging. It may be that growing older and recognising that life is shortening is the stimulus. You may be propelled by a serious illness or accident to consider living life as you would like. Perhaps problems become intolerable and you wonder if self sacrifice is worth it any more.

A time is reached where one or both do not want to continue in this way. This may occur because children are no longer dependent, retirement looms, the opportunity to study, to work outside the home, financial stability has been reached. You may simply be asking, "Is that all there is?" Growth is stimulated by crisis, when you are forced by circumstances to consider your options. This is particularly so around mid-life when you often make a major review of your life.

This was true for Elaine and Roger. They attended in crisis, Roger had had an affair, he was dissatisfied with his job, the children had left home and their sex life was non-existent. Scared for their future, unhappy with their present they did not know what to do. They were frightened of breaking up. Yet crisis can be the opportunity to breakthrough.

Travelling from childhood through early adulthood to mature adulthood is the voyage of life. Love and sex stimulate you to chart new waters. Neither in love nor troubled waters is a destination. Your relationship can take you further.

The challenge of relationship

The challenge of troubled waters is to discover what you, your self, want to change. To do this it is important to recognise how you contribute to the storms as well as your partner. This is not always easy to do for your self. Your partner may tell you what you should change but of course you will need a much broader view for both to benefit. A relationship counsellor can be most helpful. The third person on the outside can review the interaction between a couple and see the patterns of behaviour that limit each individual.

You can be a fool and not know it – but not if you are married, sums up the way you can be challenged that feels negative. A partner will in time show you all your 'faults'. This is a classic part of troubled waters.

On the positive side your partner can be a sounding board for your own ideas as you mature. The value of a relationship as an opportunity to get to know your inner self should not be overlooked. The interaction with a partner can stimulate you to emerge from the mould into which you were squeezed as a pliable child. You get to shape your self at last.

Sometimes a partner does not want you to change and resists the emergence of who you really are. 'You weren't like this when we first met', is a common rebuff. In Provisional Love you reveal only a fragment of your self. Surprisingly it can take years before you are your whole self. The distractions of work, children, TV, etc., slow down this emergence. This is a process not a static event. You continue to change your thoughts and behaviour as time alters your views and those of your beloved.

When you experience troubled waters you may be tempted to abandon ship there and then. You may decide to hang on and navigate through the storms. Unfortunately, many are likely to hang on hoping that the storm will pass. Meanwhile the love boat can sink. This is sad because it is not always necessary.

Eventually you need to address the differences that are the cause of the problems between you. It is only then that you will be clear if you desire the continuing company of each other on your voyage. Once you begin to acknowledge rather than avoid differences, you find the enthusiasm to chart new waters.

Part Four

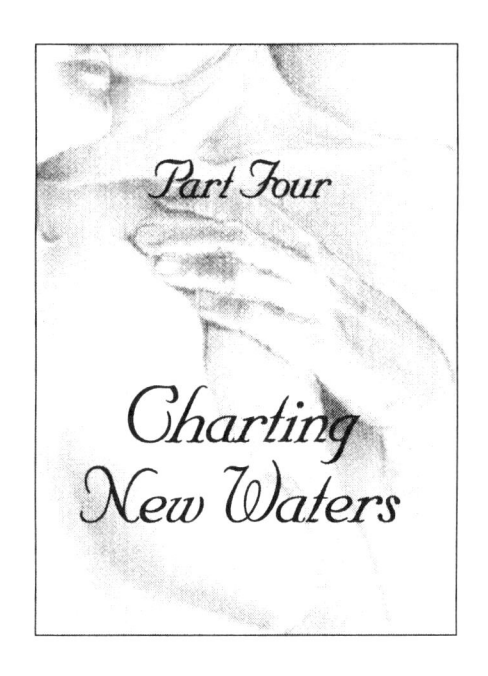

Charting New Waters

We are sailing, salty water
To be near you, to be free.

'Sailing'
Gavin Sutherland

*Maybe I have it backwards
and I'm being as big a fool as she is.
Maybe I've been waiting for her to change
and make everything alright,
when the one who needs to change is me.*

'Law of Love'
Laura Esquivel

Chapter Twelve

Changing course

Although troubled waters are unpleasant, at least you know where you are. You are still together. It takes courage to voyage beyond your usual way of behaving and thinking in the hope of navigating a better passage. In doing so you can free your selves from being swamped by unresolved problems and head into uncharted waters.

However you may be scared your situation could get worse. You may have to wait until it cannot be any worse before you change course. Many of my clients attended only when their relationship was in crisis. Then there was a lot of work to do, but also compelling reasons to chart new waters. The more stubborn you are to cling to what you know, even when you are lost at sea, the bigger the crisis it will take to awaken you. It is encouraging that more people are now seeking help or working through their own problems before they reach desperation point.

Jane and Robert (page 110) were changing course. In the counselling sessions they shared new understandings. Their insights emerged slowly over weeks of talking, writing and reading. They began to realise the part they each played in keeping their sexual problem static. Each was willing to consider how they contributed to their problem and how each could be part of breaking their established pattern. After a few sessions exploring possible reasons, things fell into place during one breakthrough session.

Robert was speaking about his first marriage. "My wife was a flirt. The marriage ended when she had an affair and left me. Jane never flirts. I feel safe when we are in company." He smiled gently at Jane.

Jane was a non-challenging partner for Robert. She was sexually shy, which in one way suited him. While Jane fell short of her sexual potential, Robert was comforted there was no risk she would have an affair. He could leave his fear of being abandoned completely undisturbed.

I asked Robert if he understood this positive aspect to their sex problem. He had not thought that any part could be positive. But this new slant did make sense to him. Robert's motive had been hidden deep in his unconcious mind. I wondered when this fear first began. It had aspects of child-like reasoning to it. Could this be a childhood learning associated with a disturbing emotion that had stuck his reasoning in the past?

"My Mum left Dad when I was eight years old. She took my sister and left me with Dad. I couldn't believe she would leave me. I felt cut off from everyone. I suppose that could contribute to my worry now." Robert's eyes opened wide.

He hit the jackpot in understanding the origin of his pattern of thinking. With his mind ticking over on this wavelength, he offered some information about Jane that he thought might be a hangover from her childhood.

"Jane has a large teddy bear collection. She plays with them sometimes. I liked this child-like part of her. She wears pretty dresses but they hide her figure. In fact I rarely see her body at all. But then no one else sees her.

"You know she really has a lovely shape. I think I'd like to see Jane wearing a fitted dress."

Although it had been no threat to be married to the safe child-like part of Jane, he also had a desire to know the woman in her.

Jane was mature in many ways. She was a graduate with a responsible job. But with Robert she could remain sexually immature and still be married. I wondered what the advantage was for her in these incongruous parts of herself. She had thoroughly discussed her early fear of sexuality associated with an episode of abuse by a family friend and no longer thought this was the major factor in her sexual reticence.

I suggested she talk about life in her family when she was a child.

"I was the eldest child of five. Mum was very sick during her last pregnancy. She never fully recovered and couldn't do much. By the time I was 9, I did most of the housework, the shopping and preparation of meals. I also took care of the younger ones. I guess I missed out on being a child."

She guessed right. She had spent much of her young life taking a mother's role and had not skipped to the delights of childhood. There was a part of Jane that yearned to play. She knew pregnancy had made her mother ill and held a fear that she might suffer the same fate. The perceived restrictions of bringing up children secretly terrified her.

At a deep level it was symbolic that she had not allowed penetration. It would mark a passage into full maturity, one that would cause her to face the possibility of motherhood. Jane's inner reluctance to be sexually mature counter-balanced Robert's fear of having a sexually active wife. They were stuck, not achieving penetration, because memories limited their desire to do so.

They realised how both had contributed to their sexual problem remaining the same over six years and began to consider new ways of being with each other. Both had to face their beliefs and update them to be relevant to their present. They each recognised the possibilities their present partner and relationship offered that was different from the past. They could choose to fix their beliefs in past learning or update their knowledge by opening their hearts to the present.

They had not been motivated at a deep level to change until a new factor made their situation intolerable. They wanted to have children but could not until intercourse became possible. Something had to change. With help they realised that the sexual block was not just about sex but involved fears from the past. They both wanted to update their learning in these areas. They both needed to trust themselves to relate to each in a way that was relevant to the present.

"*Robert is such a kind person in everything. He treats me so gently. He's never pressed me to have intercourse. I can curl up next to him and feel safe.*"

Jane clasped her hands into her chest.

"*But I can see that doesn't get us anywhere. I do want to have intercourse. I never realised part of me didn't. Now I understand I think I would like to make some changes.*"

Jane had realised the impact her childhood experience was still making on her adult life. She decided to reassess her beliefs. She was now willing to explore her own body.

"*I set aside some time, put on my favourite relaxation music, took off my clothes and lay back on the bed. I practiced some imagery which focused on relaxing while naked. It felt funny at first. Part of me thought it was wrong to touch myself. I've wanted to use tampons for ages but I just couldn't. Now I was willing to try. At first I couldn't get one in. I felt anxious but I persisted. I listened to the music some more and gently pushed it in. I was proud of myself.*"

Jane continued to relax on her own and get used to touching her genitals. When she was able to imagine herself enjoying intercourse, she felt ready to involve Robert. On his part, Robert encouraged Jane to open her eyes during sexual play and look at him. It helped them both stay in the present. She became more self assured and would tell him when she felt sexy. To help achieve penetration Robert suggested that Jane hold his erect penis at the entrance to her vagina, for as long as she wanted. He stopped moving his body away from her the instant she was uncomfortable and just stayed quietly in that position. She had the power to proceed or stop if she wanted. Gradually she was able to venture further.

Several weeks later I received a greetings card which is still in my box of treasures:

We did it!
Many thanks – Jane and Robert.

I let out a triumphant 'Yes' for them and for me. To see two people grow during therapy is the reward of the profession.

Considering change

For six years both Jane and Robert had hoped the other would make a change that would result in their having intercourse. Once they individually realised their own contribution to the problem and accepted personal responsibility, they moved forward.

Could it be you need to do the same? It is easy to think of the changes you wish your partner would make. But lasting improvement, in any situation, rests on what alteration **you** make. This does not mean that transformation is all your responsibility but it does mean that it is within your power. If you wait for your partner to change, you give up your power. That is when you feel that everything is beyond your control.

You may try trading superficial changes in behaviour, e.g., I'll agree to sit and talk about a problem – if you agree to sex. This kind of 'change' is never maintained. It is a deal done to get something in return. Only when you want to talk or have sex – in your heart and mind – is there any hope of change persisting. Long-term adjustment requires a change in perspective.

Real change rather than temporary change requires insight into your own reasons for behaving or thinking in a certain way. In a relationship if such understanding is a two-way flow, there is empathy. You each become willing to understand your own view and that of your partner.

Obviously this is much easier if you are both able to talk about and share your life experiences. As you open your mind to understand each other's different ways you have the opportunity to update your own childhood learning. You may find new respect for each other and your relationship blossoms. If the effort is one-sided the feeling of banging your head against a brick wall can be painful.

Even when you completely understand why you have developed a pattern of behaviour you cannot expect change to occur overnight. You have 20, 30 or 40 years experience of doing it your way. You may have the update clear in your conscious mind but your unconscious has years of memory of the old way. It needs retraining.

One method is to try as often as you can to do or think of the new way. Be realistic, accept that sometimes you will forget. As soon as you recognise that you have slipped back into the old pattern, stop. Then acknowledge to your self what you are doing – and if anyone else is involved tell them too. Then try again using your new way. This will retrain your unconscious until you do it automatically. Do you remember learning on your own, to swim or play golf, etc., then a coach demonstrated a better way? Did you find it took a frustrating amount of time until the new way totally replaced the old? But it does get easier with each attempt if you feel the change is of value to you. It takes practice, practice, and more practice.

Be kind to your self – and ask your partner to be kind when you fall back into the old way. Each time you correct your self you are doing well. This correction is part of relearning. If you see your partner doing something the old way that he/she wishes to change, gently let them know.

Greg and Pauline wanted to find a new way to discuss problems which had previously resulted in Greg getting angry and Pauline giving in for peace. I asked Greg if he enjoyed getting angry.

"No. It feels terrible. Like I'm about to boil over."

I asked why he persisted. A wry smile came to Greg's face.

"It works."

Pauline sat back in her chair. She had finally understood his truth.

"You mean anger is your way to get what you want. But what about what I want? You won't get away with that. My mother let Dad do the same thing. Damn it. I'm going to do it differently."

"Pressure won't lead to sex any more. It's going to be that we both want sex or no sex."

Greg was not giving up his long held behaviour easily. He tried his old emotional blackmail.

"I suppose that means never. You're frigid."

Pauline folded her arms across her chest and sat up straight.

"It won't work Greg. We can try to sort out our problems by talking and respecting each other's view. We have a chance of feeling good together. When I feel good I don't have a problem with wanting sex. I never have."

In these few words Pauline was charting new waters.

She recognised that she:

ca   allowed Greg to manipulate her

- had accepted his view that she had no sexual desire
- 'gave in' to soothe Greg's anger
- was acting like her mother when her father became angry

She then updated her thinking and responses to:
- recognise his anger and not give into it
- decide what she wanted to do if his anger persisted
- identify his anger as belonging to him
- tell him they could talk again about a problem when he was calm
- ask why he was angry and try to understand him
- decide if she wanted to live with his anger
- accept her own view of her sexuality - that she had a healthy sexual desire when she felt good in herself
- acknowledge that she felt good when they discussed problems in a calm atmosphere

Greg was unsure that a change would be better for him so he had tried his old way again. I wondered what ancient script he was playing out from his own past.

"She sounds like my mother wanting her own way all the time. Mum would get angry and Dad would agree with her instantly. I swore I wasn't going to be henpecked like Dad and have a bossy-boots wife. I've managed to keep control of things until now. Why should I change?"

Greg had learned as a child that:
- his mother got her own way by getting angry
- his father would give in
- this was not going to happen to him

Greg was not ready to change. But he could not ignore the changes in Pauline. She had stopped thinking that he had all the power. She recognised she had some of her own. It was important that she did not misuse her newly recognised power, that would merely lead to a reversal of roles. There would still be a winner and a loser.

I talked with Greg about updating his own skills for dealing with differences.

I suggested he:
- recognise his own anger
- take responsiblity to ask himself why he was angry
- share his reasons with Pauline
- thought before he acted even if he felt angry
- accept she was not going to give in
- decide for himself what views and desires he valued.
- did not have to behave like his father or mother, only himself

Neither Greg's parents nor Pauline's had worked out how to live respectfully in harmony. Both sets of parents had troubled relationships. They in turn had learned their patterns from their parents. Greg and Pauline needed some new skills to discuss respectfully - ones they had not learned in childhood.

Their parents did what they could in an era when even talking about marital distress was met with disapproval from others. Using the help available Greg and Pauline wanted to relate in a different way to their parents.

A word of caution

If you have had a pattern of giving in to anger and decide to stop doing this, it is necessary for your safety to consider if your partner would endanger you physically. If you sense he/she would harm you if you stand firm you can choose to remove your self from the source of anger.

If this seems a fearful choice there are support agencies and counsellors you can contact. The excellent book *Emotional Blackmail*[15] further explores how to stop manipulation in a relationship.

However, angry pressure is often only exerted while it is effective. Pauline was beginning to realise this. She was ready to update her thinking and behaviour. Greg could also consider his behaviour in a new light. Could they cope with respectful discussion? Time would tell.

Respectful discussion

It is common that two people have a different way to deal with a problem. You may feel responsible to solve the problem for your partner (often a masculine style). Or you just want to be heard while you voice your dilemma (often a feminine style).

Whatever your style, it is important to realise initially you each have a limited view of the problem – your own. You each think what you would do to resolve the problem. If you offer suggestions early on your partner may not feel heard. It is likely that your suggestions are appropriate for you but not your partner. Patience is required whilst you listen and attempt to understand what the problem means to the other.

Inability to resolve problems is the most common cause of marital disharmony. In fact, not only in marriage do you encounter this difficulty but in all relationships – at work, with parents, children, friends, shop assistants, other car drivers, etc. At the extreme of inability to resolve problems lies war. People with different political, cultural or religious ideas become irreconcilable. Sometimes living with a beloved can feel like living in a war zone.

Why is harmony so difficult? The basic cause lies in beliefs that are entrenched and limit your options. You may slip into 'I am right, he/she is wrong'. From this position you are in the contest to win. The usual outcome is a winner and a loser. The original problem has not been solved and continues in some shape or form. This had been the situation for Greg and Pauline. Until they attended for counselling their differences of opinion followed a fixed path. Greg would get angry and yell. It was clear to Greg that Pauline was wrong.

Pauline would either complain about his behaviour, walk away and not speak to him for days, or give in. It was clear to Pauline that Greg was wrong.

The techniques they used included:
- blaming
- yelling
- threatening
- complaining
- walking away
- giving in

Not one of these is a problem solving technique. They are all avoidance techniques. It is possible to work through problems. If you choose to do this, you can reach either a respectful settlement or the recognition that the beliefs of each are fundamentally different. The latter can be scary because it requires that you will be separate on this issue.

When you are different you do not receive the reinforcement that your partner agrees with you. Your ego is not boosted. But uncovering of difference rather than false agreement does wonders for self esteem. As differences are appreciated between your self and your beloved, you can assess how important they are to you. This is vital to the nature of the relationship – the basis of which is honest relating.

Before trying out some new ways I suggested that Greg and Pauline consider some:

Golden Rules for respectful discussion

- Have a basic respect for the other person.
- Have respect for your own views.
- Consider both views have value.
- Allow that you each deserve an equal opportunity to express your view.

- Allow time to listen to each other.
- Listen with your ears and mind open – your mouth closed!
- Be honest about your ideas and feelings.
- Say what you think.
- Do not alter what you say to try to please your partner.
- State what you feel and think using 'I' statements ('You' is often a criticism).
- Establish a safe climate – no threats, no pressure.
- Hang in. Do not withdraw into silence, tears, criticism.
- Not expect the other to read your mind.
- Put your self in the position of the other to try to understand their view.
- Look for the common ground.
- Hear and assess new information.
- Know it is healthy to be able to decide to remain with your opening opinion or to adjust your view.
- Allow time.

As you read these rules you will realise that trying to resolve a problem takes time.

Raising a problem when your partner is rushing out of the door is an attempt to gain an unfair advantage. You may get a quick solution but not resolve the problem adequately.

With these Golden Rules in mind, Pauline and Greg attempted to find out how their weekend argument could change to respectful discussion. Greg began:

"I want to go fishing. You never want to go so I suppose I'll have to go on my own."

Greg had said what he wanted. That was a good start. Then he blew it by trying to make Pauline feel guilty in his you statement. I suggested he try again. Greg twitched his nose and drew in a breath:

"I would like to go fishing today. I'd enjoy your company if you want to come along."

By George, he's got it!

Pauline responded:

"I'd like to come along but the garden needs weeding. Couldn't you help with that?"

Pauline now tried to manipulate Greg with her you statement. I suggested she try again and say what she wanted to do that weekend. I encouraged her to state any concerns she had.

"I want to do some study this weekend. I want to spend some time with you. I am bothered that the garden needs weeding. I don't know how to do it all." Pauline let out a relieved sigh.

There was some common ground – they wanted to spend some time together. They also had different wants to discuss. They re-read the 'Golden Rules for respectful discussion'.

Greg continued:

"I realise the garden is a mess but I don't want to spend the whole weekend working. I've had a busy week and I'm tired. It would do me good to relax and go fishing. Sounds like you need some time to study. How can we sort this out?"

I could sense Greg feeling good using his discussion skills rather than arguing. Greg had acknowledged Pauline's concern about the garden and her need to study. He had equally acknowledged his own need to relax.

He told Pauline how he felt. He did not offer a solution but had offered to continue looking at the problem. Pauline had more enthusiasm to talk further when she was not distracted by anger. She could face their dilemma. She felt good in Greg's company. Now she wanted to spend time with him. As their feelings improved they both got into the swing of respectful discussion.

"If we put a chair in the car, I could pack my books and sit and study while you fish. As long as you don't interrupt me while I study. It would be good to be out of the house in the fresh air.

"How would you feel about weeding tomorrow?"

Pauline was asking Greg how he felt rather than trying to manoeuvre him.

"Not too keen. I don't like gardening. But I know it needs doing, so OK. Maybe we should think about a house with a smaller garden or pay someone to help. We are too busy to maintain this one." Greg invitingly opened his hands.

Greg had made a healthy adjustment. He had considered all the factors affecting his time over the weekend. He also did not want to continue making the compromise of caring for a garden when his free time was limited. He suggested a change, to reduce the burden of gardening.

Both had shifted from their original view. Without the anxiety of the war zone their minds were able to conceive new ideas. The outcome was they both felt good.

But there may have been other factors that affected their discussion.

Pauline may have preferred to study at home. Then each would have to choose what was important – to be together that afternoon or to follow their pursuits separately.

If a couple find that they have no interests to share they may spend a lot of time separately. Each must then decide how much companionship they want in their relationship.

How does this way of discussing a difference compare to the previous style of win/lose? How many times would you enter win/lose before giving up on a problem (and on your partner)? Do you think respectful discussion is worth the time and effort?

The differences to consider are:

Win/lose conflict

Rules

closed minds
blame
not listening fully
expectations of the other
lack of understanding for the opposite view
trying to get the other to agree with you
rapid or pressured end
not revealing all you feel

Results

confusion
anger
argument
at least one person feels bad
problem remains unresolved

'Resolutions'

give in

walk away
unhealthy compromise with heavy heart

Respectful discussion

Rules

open minds
neither is wrong
ears and heart open
let go of expectations
put your self in the other's shoes
respect for difference

time, no pressure
open honesty

Results

clarity
interest
discussion
two people feel good
resolution

Resolutions

agree to disagree
– act separately
agreement.
healthy adjustment with a light heart

Greg had been patient during much of the talking, but he could not contain his frustration any longer. He wanted some action.

He threw his arms in the air.

"This is all very fine, but how does this help sort out our sex problem?"

This was the first time Greg had used 'our' rather than 'her' to define the problem with sex. I thought he could now answer his own question. I asked him to think which situation - argument or respectful discussion - was most likely to stir sexual desire.

"When I get frustrated sexually that leads to me getting angry. My urge is satisfied if we have sex. But I don't enjoy sex as much as I do when Pauline is interested. Anyway, she told me my anger won't work anymore. The peaceful afternoon at the river could have a better chance, I suppose. We'll have to try and see what happens."

Greg was still unsure but he did reveal a change of perspective. Pauline was definite:

"The river sounds good. I felt warm towards Greg as we talked just then. He didn't put me down. He didn't yell. If it was always like that I'd feel like sex. I don't want sex when he's angry, though I have given in to get him off my back. But that's in the past."

This may sound simple but to make and then maintain a change takes effort. Over the next few months, Greg and Pauline had more arguments. They had ongoing stresses in their lives. But gradually the arguments became less severe. In the midst of a quarrel, Pauline or Greg would at some stage realise that they were back on their old non-productive path and call a halt. They would then agree to talk when both had calmed down. Their effort was supported by the good feelings that flowed from respectful discussion.

They both had individual therapy to help break their old patterns of anger and appeasement learned from their parents. They also began to make some changes in the demands of the lifestyle they had been hooked into. They worked together on a budget for their expenditure and planned to move to a less expensive house with a small garden.

Greg realised that he had been pushing himself to please everyone else. He had grown up with a Protestant work ethic which he had never thought to question. When he did, he chose to update this belief and decided he had gone over the top with work. Greg reduced his hours in his business.

He found when he was calmer he could work more efficiently. With less stress he was less needy of sexual relief and more interested in sexual sharing.

Pauline continued her studies. She felt less stressed and found that she could concentrate better. She began to reclaim her self respect. She also respected Greg's efforts, realising how difficult change was for him.

As respect returned to their relating, sexual desire re-emerged in Pauline. They did have a different level of sex drive, but they now realised their levels of desire were far closer than either would have thought possible. Calling on their new respectful discussion skills Greg and Pauline achieved a new perspective on sex.

Starting with an old scenario they worked out a new way. Greg and Pauline summarised their old style for dealing with 'No'. I asked them to note their feelings. Then they considered how they could update their thinking and behaviour and how this felt. Their efforts are clear in the next table:

When one says 'No'

Old style:

Greg

I ask if she wants sex.
I get angry.
I tell her she is frigid.
I keep asking until she says 'Yes'.

Feelings at end
Empty, not appreciated.

Pauline
I watch TV until he is asleep to avoid sex.
I say I'm tired.
I turn my back on him.
I tell him he's obsessed.
I agree, to keep him quiet.

Dead, unloved.

Updated style:

Greg
I tell her I feel sexy.

I won't put her down
- ('You're frigid').
If I feel angry, I'll think about why.

I'll talk when I calm down inside.
Does 'No' mean there is a problem?
I feel sad when you turn away.
I feel close when I touch you.
Sometimes I feel really horny.

If you don't I can masturbate.
I enjoy sex when we both feel it's right.

Pauline
I tell him on this occasion I don't.
I won't make up excuses.
I'll watch TV when I want
- but not to avoid sex.
I won't put him down - ('You're obsessed').
If he tells me he's angry. I'll say, 'I can see that, I am responsible for how I behave right now but that's for you to sort out.'
Trust myself not to give in because he's angry.
If there's a problem I'll talk about it
- not wait for sex before I do.
When you say how you feel, I want to face you.
That feels good.
So do I but not always at the same time as you.
That's your choice.

I feel the same.

Feelings at end
Not so bad.

Respected and loved.

This way of relating felt better to Greg and Pauline. It involved a new approach. The more they discussed issues with respect and honesty the more they found they could accept 'No' or 'Yes' without need for justification. You will see their style gradually evolved even further as they reached mature love (Chapter Sixteen).

Does their new style of relating suit you? The best guide is to check how you feel at each step when discussing a difference.

Stay true to your self, then you can be sure the new course you chart is the one you want to follow.

I found the greatest love of all inside of me,
Learning to love your Self is the greatest love of all.

'The Greatest Love of All'
Michael Masser, Linda Creed

Chapter Thirteen

Becalmed

There are times when a best friend may seem to understand you better than your beloved. But when differences arise with a friend you can walk away thus avoiding any conflict. This is not the best option aboard the love boat as you have seen in the previous chapters through Pauline and Greg, Robert and Jane. Instead, you learn how to discuss difference, with respect, as a result of sharing the storms of relationship. Relieved you are leaving troubled waters in your wake you may linger in the calm but as you gaze out across the vast ocean you may wonder 'where to from here'? Free to express your self with your partner you begin to explore the uncharted depths of your own potential. If you are tempted to tarry too long in the calm, love and sex will awaken you to continue your voyage.

Respect for difference

You may yearn for your loved one to agree with you on everything but you know this occurs only in dreams. A real relationship, however, can still flourish, without complete agreement, based on healthy respect for difference. If it feels good in your heart to be with your partner, then do it. If you reach this decision with joy you have not compromised your self. You have chosen a partner in whose presence you can continue to grow.

A relationship can accommodate being separate and being together. To do this check during each situation if you feel joyful with your choice. A heavy heart is a sure sign that you are pleasing someone else but not your self. When you feel a heavy heart review your choice and be willing to have the courage to follow the right course for you.

You can find individual pleasure in pursuing a different interest separate from your partner. When you return to each other's company you can share your enthusiasm with joy. You can obtain the delightful balance of separateness and sharing.

Fundamental difference

However, sometimes there is such a fundamental difference between two people that following their heart's desire sets them on divergent courses. David and Susan were not sure why they were arguing, but a fundamental difference underlay their conflicts. They had managed to side step a subject of major importance for the eight years they had been living together. In this way they had lived harmoniously but recently they had begun to argue at the slightest provocation. This was such a change and made no sense to them. To help unravel their confusion they completed the questionnaire, Positive signals for continuing, from 'in love', (page 108). David and Susan appeared well suited, each scoring around 20. I noticed on their questionnaire that Susan had answered 'No' to 'discussed big issues such as children, finance, etc.'.

David disagreed. "We have talked about all of those."

Susan thought differently. "Yes we have talked but we haven't agreed to have children."

This was one gigantic issue that had not been resolved.

"I have always wanted children, David didn't. But it didn't seem too important. I thought with time he'd come round. Whenever we talked about children we would come up with good reasons for delay. He wanted to get established in his career. Then we decided to take some overseas trips, which we both enjoyed. But now I am 34 and I feel I can't put off a decision any longer. It isn't normal not to want kids."

In Susan's view it was not normal. But for David it was. He was very definite:

"I don't want children. I'm not frightened to have kids. I like them but I like our life with its freedom even more. I don't want the responsibility of child-raising."

Over eight years they had both valued their relationship and grown. But now the reality of their present indicated they needed to move on. They each revealed a fundamental part of themselves that was different. It could not be negotiated. You either have children or you do not. For either to change their view would have compromised their fundamental desire. All the love and liking in the world could not keep these two together. They decided to part so that each could have the opportunity to fulfil an essential part of happiness. At the time of separation there are two approaches you can adopt to resolve a situation that is difficult for both:

1. With respect.

You can honour the love you have known. You move on with sadness for the loss but recognise that you must each follow your own path. Gentle but clear words allow each to move on − 'I'll miss you but I need to be separate. I can't fulfil this part of me with you.'

2. With disrespect.

You can dishonour the love you have known with vindictiveness, punishment or intimidation. Angry words and threats to control the other are attempts to prevent someone from following their heart −

'I'll make sure you get nothing.' 'My solicitor will get you.' 'I'll kill you.' 'I'll kill myself.'

David and Susan chose to honour their years together. Using respectful discussion they reached a fair financial settlement. Within two years they had both married other people.

Susan married a man who was busting to start a family. They now have two children. David married a career woman, aged 42, who had also made a definite choice not to have children. David and Susan have remained friends.

If you choose the second option of win/lose, things can get very nasty. Divorce lawyers have many unpleasant tales to tell. The movie, 'The War of the Roses', took this to the ultimate extreme. The battle between husband and wife ended with them killing each other. Even if you do not go to this ultimate end, emotional and financial pain often result. There is a better way. David and Susan found it.

If you find your self in this situation but settlement is proving hard to achieve there are professional mediation services[16] that can assist you. The counsellors are skilled in using a respectful approach, which can result in the fairest settlement for both.

Why do we find it difficult to automatically discuss with respect?

There seem to be two important underlying obstacles to overcome:

1. A culture of win/lose.

This is the remnant of a society still attached to the animal model of the survival of the fittest. Originally based on competition between the physically strong and the weak, it has led to much human suffering. We have always lived with conflict between people of different ideas and different philosophies, yet human compassion can allow you to treat others as equals. It leads you to the more sophisticated and satisfying human experience of respect.

2. A culture of Self-flagellation.

I am not talking about masochistic sexual stimulation. But of a culture that refers to 'Self' in many derogatory ways. How often have you been told (or tell your Self) you are – self-indulgent, selfish or self-centred when you are simply stating what you want (when another wants something different). How much kinder could you be to your Self if you thought in terms of Self-caring, being your Self or Self-assured. Such thoughts form the basis of that highly desirable attribute – Self-esteem.

What is Self with a capital 'S'?

What is Self? Where does it come from? When does Self come into existence? Did you have knowledge, feelings, personality from your beginning or become your Self later as you absorbed lessons from older people?

No one can provide absolute proof to substantiate answers to these questions, though everyone has an opinion. Self has been viewed as spirit or soul by religion – the mind, by psychology – and as genetic inheritance by science. However you personally conceive the exact nature of Self, you will be aware that we each have an individual essence, as unique as our fingerprints.

Born as a bundle of joy you gradually develop not as one Self but two. The first, your original, loving, inner Self is the one designated a capital 'S'.

The second, your outer self only rates a small 's' because it is not original and develops in response to the standards of others. This outer self becomes the armour coat you wear to survive in the community. Unfortunately, it but may also act as a barrier between your inner Self and intimate connection with another.

This dual nature of self/Self in one person leads to all kinds of frustration in life, particularly in personal relationships. To be your authentic, integrated and joyous whole Self you will need to 'sort your Self out'! For many, living life only through their outer self lies at the heart of their problems in love and sex.

Being your Self versus selfish

Elaine and Roger desperately wanted to 'sort them selves out'. One of the facets of Self they struggled to understand was the difference between being selfish and being your Self. They were not sure there was any difference.

"Doing what pleases me is being myself. I can be myself with my friends. But I can't with Roger."

Elaine lowered her eyes to the floor as she said the final sentence.

"Selfish is when you set out to do something to hurt someone - to get what you want at their expense. But you have to give and take in a relationship. You can't have what you want if the other objects," Roger reasoned.

Roger had started his definition of selfish with the awareness of bad intent towards someone else. But then he sacrificed his Self to focus on what another wanted, as more important than his own desire.

"If it makes Roger unhappy when I do what I want – that's selfish. I don't want to hurt him. I love him. If he's happy there's no harm."

Elaine loved Roger but not her own inner Self. Her definition that selfish - when your partner (or parent) does not approve of what you do but you do it anyway - was the very essence of losing her Self. How a partner feels when you state what you want is their responsibilty - not yours.

Elaine tried to second guess how Roger would respond before saying what she wanted. Trying to decide whether what you want is acceptable to someone else leads to a terrible knot of confusion. This can be cleared by asking your self these questions:

Am I being my Self or selfish?

                                            Yes   No   Don't know

1. Am I setting out to hurt him/her?
2. Am I treating my Self as equal?
3. Am I setting out to win at all costs?
4. Am I being respectful of another?
5. Am I taking advantage of him/her?
6. Am I honouring my Self?

'Yes' to 2, 4 and 6 are essentials in being your Self.

'Yes' to questions 1, 3 and 5 knowingly disregards the value of another. That is selfish.

Answering 'Don't know' is a sure sign of losing contact with your Self.

You may find it easier to answer these questions if they are related to situations connected with work, interests, sport, etc., but find this questionnaire to be much more difficult to answer when in the setting of your love relationship.

Self awareness

When the basics of life for the community, safety, food and shelter are scarce it is necessary for the common good to override individual desires. As the basics of life become secure, individuality can emerge. In the developed world we have reached this stage and we have entered an era of Self awareness. The community is still important but the values of your community are changing. When you value your Self and thus find happiness from the inside, the community benefits from your positive contribution.

Losing touch with your inner Self

Self sacrifice as the right way to be, has been promoted by some religions. The impression is given that if your life is a struggle now, providing no joy in this present, rewards will be gained in heaven. You hope at least to be respected and appreciated by others for your struggles. But there is a difference between struggle and effort. Struggle is to do something that offends your spirit. You may obtain a material reward, but the happiness generated is short lived. Effort is to work with dedication at something that brings inner pleasure in the here and now and continues to do so.

Every time you check with others as to how you should be, you misplace your self. If you hide part of your self to win admiration, you may gain their approval but you pay the heaviest price – you lose touch with your inner Self.

Do you think, 'If I don't do what pleases him/her, I might lose him/her?' If you apply this type of logic you may indeed avoid 'losing' the other. But the concept that you can lose someone else results from the assumption that you own their love in the first place. In sacrificing your Self to obtain the love of another you may well expect he/she should appreciate your sacrifice. But often another resents the trade-off, realising that much is due in return. He/she becomes aware of the burden of pleasing to be pleased and seek their freedom. That is when you really 'lose' someone.

It takes many years to lose contact with your inner Self. The process begins at an early age when you learn to Self sacrifice to win approval from parents, teachers, peers. They learned this pattern from their loved ones. But the times they are a changing. We are living longer than ever before. We are more financially independent than ever before, at least for basic needs such as food and shelter. This presents the exciting opportunity to mature to reach full potential in a way that was not available to previous generations fearful of war, poverty and the disgrace of being alone. It is possible to find fulfilment in a way that is not greedy but is fuelled by love for your Self and others.

If you challenge the doctrine of Self sacrifice and release your Self, a sense of relief can enter your life. You can experience feeling good, exploring the world of the senses, feelings and thinking from your own inner base, not as a reflection of the experiences of others.

Self sacrifice can be held up as a virtue. But when it leads to resentment, anger or unhappiness this 'virtue' is worthy of deeper examination. What are your deeply held values? Do you Self sacrifice or Self care? This questionnaire will make the difference clearer.

Self care or Self sacrifice?

Yes   No   Sometimes

1. Am I doing what is right for me?
2. Am I caring for my health?
3. Am I responsible for his/her feelings?
4. Do I say what I want?
5. Do I feel resentful when I compromise?
6. I worry if my partner will love me if I do/say what I prefer.
7. Do I say 'No' when I don't want sex?
8. Am I open and honest with my partner?
9. Do I give in for peace?
10. Do I please to win approval?

Answering 'Yes' to 1, 2, 4, 7 and 8 is evidence of Self care. These are also part of your Self esteem.

If you said 'Yes' to 3, 5, 6, 9 and 10, these are examples of Self sacrifice. These are the areas in which you could consider an update of past learning to improve Self esteem in your present.

Could it be that when you answer 'sometimes' these are the times you lose your Self?

Releasing your Self

How do you release your inner Self when it has been partly hidden for much of your life? There are critical times in your life during which strong emotion or deep questioning of values, allow your Self to be raised to consciousness. You become aware that you are not living as your true Self but as a reflection of others. Perhaps all others see is your outer self. You become miserable, even depressed, when you accept that the armour suit of your outer self is your all.

You may first glimpse your self mirrored in the eyes of a beloved who shines back your best features. Roger had known this early on with Elaine but over the years she also reflected back some of his less wonderful qualities. His Self esteem was low when he met Barbara. Briefly he gained esteem reflected from Barbara.

"Elaine used to be interested in my paintings but not now. I was losing interest in painting until Barbara came along. She was full of praise and I felt really great."

Roger was relaxed during a session on his own.

Roger was looking for a boost to his esteem, via his painting, from another. But he needed to tap into a more sustainable source of esteem from his inner Self. He thought his work was good when someone else praised it, without that he was unsure of the value of his creative work, which originated in his Self.

"I met Barbara at the theatre group. We found we shared an interest in art. I asked her to look at my work. I valued her opinion. Barbara was very knowledgeable about art. She admired my paintings. We talked a lot. One thing led to another and we had an affair. I didn't plan it that way.

"She was so enthusiastic about my paintings, though I thought they were ordinary. You know pretty gum trees that everyone likes.

"Being with Barbara I felt a new excitement. I began to paint all

the ideas that I'd had in my head but could never express within the limits of teaching. My style began to change. Barbara wasn't keen on the more expressive paintings I was doing. I became unwilling to show her my latest painting as she was critical. I wanted to show her but what if she didn't like it? Some I'd face to the wall. I showed her only the paintings I knew she would like. I noticed the type of painting she admired. I painted some in that style. But I became dissatisfied with my painting. It lost its joy. Instead of being passionate about my painting I became depressed feeling untalented. I lost my enthusiasm.

"I noticed she didn't want to make love with me. I still felt very passionate towards her. In the end she left me. I felt cheated I had bared my soul to her, shown her my Self. I didn't want to lose her. I was willing to do whatever she wanted. But she left. I allowed myself to be vulnerable and I got hurt. I felt like I did when I was a child."

Roger had lost contact with his Self during his marriage to Elaine. The exuberant feelings he had in the affair with Barbara released the creative part of his Self. Buoyed by her regard, he felt wonderful. When she no longer offered approval his inner Self went back into hiding. He was repeating the pattern that he had developed as a child when his mother or father did not approve. He repeated the same pattern as an adult with Elaine and then Barbara.

You can try to deny or repress your inner Self but it is made of strong stuff and keeps niggling away telling you to pay it sufficient notice. If you ignore this irritating inner voice it will reach consciousness some other way, at the least as a sensation of mild discontent or as seriously as depression. Or the dis-ease may present in the body as physical symptoms such as muscle tightness, headaches, irritable bowel or indigestion. More serious illnesses such as cancer and heart disease have also been linked with continued inner distress.

You may be stimulated to take a new look at life by a close encounter with mortality, when someone close to you dies. Other distressing major life events such as a serious illness, financial loss, divorce, or children leaving home may release your inner life force to rise to the surface demanding that you pay attention to your Self.

This important stage in life has been called the **'mid-life crisis'**. Crisis is vital for change as we are fairly comfortable to ignore our Self until a sizeable challenge means we need to tap into our inner strength. In response you may opt to do no more than recycle the past but in a new setting.

A new partner, a new location, a new job may temporarily quieten your inner Self to stop pestering you. If you choose one of these but have made no changes in your thinking you will be faced with other challenges in the future and have to go through the whole process again. Your inner Self demands attention until you take heed.

If crisis forces you to listen to your own wisdom you can grow to experience the release of the **'mid-life transition'**. There is one vital question, which is evoked at this time. If you consider it carefully it can turn a crisis into transition:

Who am I?

Your dual natured self/Self is confronted by this question. You will need some time to answer this. You may like to close your eyes and hear the words that first come to mind about your self when you ask:

Who am I?

Now write down the words you used about your self
'I am..,'
Did you include any of the following?
I am ....   a mother/father
                     a daughter/son

married/single/divorced
a nurse, bricklayer, etc. (the job I do)

or

where you live
the number of children you have
my hobby is............
my body is, e.g., fat/thin, hair colour, tall/short
I own a car........., etc.

These are descriptions of your present role in life and your possessions. They are descriptions of the outer self. The reference for each of these is external. They are a statement of: what you do, what you have, the body armour in which you carry your Self. You have not revealed who you are – on the inside.

Have another attempt to describe who you are. This time – from the inside, without reference to any one else.

Again you may increase your focus by closing your eyes and taking a series of deep breaths.

What words came to mind this time? Did they include such descriptions as :

'I am.............................'

    kind
    loving
    creative
    fun
    thoughtful
    stimulated by life
    intelligent
    optimistic
    compassionate

If you have not asked your inner Self, 'Who am I?' ever before, you may at first respond 'I don't know'. Caught in the performance of life's actions you may not know your inner Self – yet.

You may revisit this question many times in your life before you know your Self fully and feel at ease.

∼

Becalmed

*After a while you learn the subtle difference
between holding a hand and chaining a soul.
And you learn that love does not mean leaning
and company does not mean security.
And you begin to learn that kisses are not contracts
and presents are not promises.
And you begin to accept a refusal
with your head up and your eyes clear
with the grace of an adult,
not the heartache of a child.*

Author unknown

Chapter Fourteen

The wind in your sails

You are getting to know your Self better. You are awakening and your inner strength has become the wind in your sails. You know the direction you want to take. However, this time of personal growth can also be confusing for you and your partner. You originally thought you knew each other well and now you realise there is much more to learn. You may well have different thoughts about the course you want to set but do you both desire to reach the shores of the heart together? How do you stay true to your Self, and share the love boat?

Initially, the changes you make may send your boat off in one direction then another. At first you are dependent your partner for approval. Finally, you may decide to express your own heartfelt wants but find this difficult. In desperation you grab hold of the wheel and swing hard over to declare your independence yelling, 'I'll do what I want and you can go to Hell!' Suddenly there is a man or woman overboard.

Do you want to set sail on your own or when your partner has had a swim around; do you want to invite him/her to climb aboard as a companion on the voyage?

If you find you are unable to be your Self with your partner you may be the one who jumps ship, fleeing from a loved one to obtain your independence.

Independence

Pauline was struggling in this way.

"Generally things are going pretty well. But I still find it hard to do what I want with Greg. I can do it now with the children and with my friends. But with Greg I find myself still agreeing with him even when I don't want to. I can't believe I do this after all the therapy we've been through. I suppose it's the old me, giving in for peace. It would be easier to separate, then I could be independent. I'd be able to do whatever I want."

Pauline would have found it easier to be her Self on her own. Leaving Greg would bring instant relief from her dilemma but eventually she would have to face her tendency to give in. It was her pattern of behaviour even more than the way Greg responded that she needed to change. Until she did this she would not know her Self nor would she know Greg.

I wondered if she could recall a recent, specific instance where she had not expressed her true opinion.

"Greg spends a lot of money on electronic stuff for his photographic system. Every new thing that comes out he has to have. A new camera, computer imaging, scanner, you name it he buys it. He tells me about each new invention and explains why he needs to buy it. Then he asks me if I agree. At the moment I don't. The washing machine is not working well and I think we should spend the money on a new one.

"He says he works hard to earn the money and it's his relaxation and the washing machine will keep going for a while longer. I say OK. He buys his new addition and is happy and relaxed. I know we talked about his level of stress and photography does help him relax. But I have

to keep mopping up the laundry floor where the machine leaks each time I use it.

"I don't think he's being understanding of what I want. If I was on my own I'd have a new washing machine, not an extra bit for a camera."

On her own Pauline would have an easy decision. But she would not learn to value her wants as equal to Greg's. I asked her to respect both their desires and talk to Greg.

"I've tried talking to Greg but we can't agree on this. If I was taking care of myself I would buy a new washing machine. I think it is a priority. Greg could either wait or sell one of the cameras he no longer uses."

I wondered what was stopping her from buying the machine.

"I'd feel guilty. Greg earns the money so I feel he decides how it is spent."

She was not valuing her own contribution to the marriage as equal.

I suggested she try doing what she wanted. She was already thinking of leaving to find the freedom to make her own decisions. Why not make one in the marriage and see what happened? At the worst they would separate as a result but there may be other outcomes. She decided she had nothing to lose.

She returned to see me two weeks later.

"I couldn't believe it. I spoke to Greg again. I told him it was important for me to buy the washing machine. I said it was his decision about the camera. I bought the machine the next day. He was stunned when it was delivered. But then he surprised me. He advertised his previous model camera in the newspaper. He sold it for a few hundred dollars and paid for the new equipment he wanted. I felt free to do something for myself. Greg said he felt good not having to ask me what he could buy."

Did she still feel like separating?

"I don't want to leave. I respected how Greg took responsibility for his purchase. I respected myself. I now feel excited that I can be independent and be married to Greg."

Independence on your own is certainly a pendulum swing away from dependence. However, if the fear of non-acceptance remains, isolation and loneliness can result if you withdraw into independence. Overcoming this fear presents the opportunity to be your Self whoever else is around. If you desire a partner, you will find balance lies in maintaining your independence in their presence. You experience this joyous freedom by being open and honest with your partner.

When you follow the direction of your own wisdom you gain the courage for your outer self to be the same as your inner Self. Not just on your own but in any company. You find pleasure relates to knowing what you want, respecting the wants of others, but ultimately choosing for your Self what you will do.

A relationship in which you remain true to your Self and respect another can be nourishing to the welfare of both individuals. The term 'interdependence' is used to describe this sustaining connection.

Interdependence

Interdependence means to be your Self and share with respect for another. No Self sacrifice is required because you no longer need approval. You know who you are and are willing to let another see all of you – inside and out. The more significant the relationship, the more Self esteem is required to maintain your Self in company.

When you live true to your Self you can show your friends, lover and respected colleagues, your whole person. If they, in response, choose you and offer the same openness, you make a respectful connection. Even when you do not agree with each other, you meet in respect.

The effort to emerge as your Self is rewarded with Self esteem. With Self respect you can face that another may not choose you. You no longer need everyone to like you because you like your Self. It is better to recognise whom you do not like and who does not like your true Self. You avoid the heartache of forging a relationship that will not nourish either.

Susan and David (page 206) eventually revealed the whole of their Selves to each other. They recognised their love and it was strong enough to appreciate their fundamental difference. To fulfil their different dreams on children they chose different marital partners. They each found happiness separately and retained mutual respect.

Robert and Jane (page 110) revealed their Selves to each other. In doing so they recognised they could continue together and not compromise their desires. They found their happiness in interdependence.

You may find it surprisingly difficult to be your Self when you have not done so for years. But coming to know your Self provides the wind in your sails that will take you further on the voyage to happiness and fulfilment.

When you feel confident to say, 'what I show you is who I am,' you are revealing your true Self. When you are being your Self another can truly get to know you and choose if this is the person they like, if this is the person they share fundamental beliefs with and if this is the person with whom they wish to share some of their lifetime. This is a solid foundation for interdependence.

Relationships of love and sex seem to be the most challenging way to awaken your Self. Yet it is through this process that you can experience the fullest sense of aloneness and completeness. Emerging from troubled waters and facing the effort of charting new waters you learn not to waste the present but to enjoy the precious moments of each day on your own or shared with a beloved.

Equality in a relationship allows the desires of another to be considered equal yet not competitive – to be understood and considered with respect. If there is agreement this is obviously easy. If there is disagreement you now know a respectful discussion can occur. With Self respect you will inevitably be separate on some issues. But in the warmth of love, decisions are no longer made from fear of the response of the other, nor to win or control.

In mature love there is nothing to fear in your Self and therefore in the other. When this respect is mingled with sexual desire the combination can be dynamite.

Your Self in sex

When you live your life under your own direction you discover your talents and passions. Sharing a passionate life with another is a vital aspect of sexual desire. Sexual satisfaction is a spontaneous flow on from this.

To love each other in revealing discussion **and** revealing sex is a high achievement. He has extended his Self to open up to the pleasure of sharing his inner thoughts and feelings. She has extended her Self to open up to the pleasure of sharing and revealing her sexuality. By opening their outer selves they reach through to their inner Selves.

Each makes the connection of masculine and feminine aspects and experiences the satisfaction of completeness.

The gentle flow of feelings between two people is one of the experiences of love. The tenderness of mutual exposure of inner Selves, away from the harshness of the modern world allows you to be soft, to be kind and experience loving. The sheer joy of being alive today, here and now, is in itself wonderful. But the icing on the cake is the respectful sharing of this experience in the presence of another.

It can be a very grown-up experience when two fully mature adults share them Selves. It is not about 'what do I have to give to get' but a comfortable, respectful sharing.

Although there are challenges there is also much to be learned and enjoyed on the voyage. To love another involves being your Self, loving life and expressing that in the richest and fullest way that you can. There is something so perfectly luscious about kind respectful, loving and sexual sharing with another, the very nectar of the Gods.

You may like to consider what you have read about respectful discussion and being your Self in the light of your own sexual relationship. These questions in different sections will prompt you to identify what is happening in your relationship at present:

Honesty
- Do you make time to talk with each other?
- Can you tell your partner anything?
- Who knows most about your feelings - your partner or your best friend?
- Can you say 'No' to your partner?
- Do you know your inner Self?
- Do you know your partner?
- Do you want to know more?
- Do you have a passion?
- Do you share a passion?
- Do you like your outer self?
- Do you like your partner?

Balance
- Do you have private time?
- Can you relax - on your own?
- Can you relax in each other's company?
- Do you have fun?
- Do you like your balance between work and play?

- ❧ Do you take care of your Self?
- ❧ Do you care about others?

Behaviour
- ❧ Do you take full responsibility for your actions?
- ❧ Does your partner take full responsibility for their behaviour?
- ❧ Do you want to update any of your own behaviour?
- ❧ Do you want to expand your limits?
- ❧ Do you decide what is right for you?
- ❧ Do you like your behaviour?
- ❧ Do you like your partner's behaviour?
- ❧ Do you take time to talk?

Discussion
- ❧ Does your partner listen to your problems?
- ❧ Can you easily discuss problems with your partner?
- ❧ Do you listen?
- ❧ Do you try to understand your own views?
- ❧ Do your try to understand your partner's views?
- ❧ Do you go through problems or around them?
- ❧ Can you cope with disappointment gracefully?

Equality
- ❧ Do you feel that household tasks are fairly distributed?
- ❧ Does your partner consider your view in matters that affect you both?
- ❧ Do you consider his/her views?
- ❧ Do you talk together about important concerns?
- ❧ Do you think you are right he/she is wrong?
- ❧ Do you have a system of sharing finances that suits you both?

Sex and Love
- ❧ Is sex as good or better than when you were first together?

- Are you fulfilled when you have sex?
- Do you enjoy sex now?
- Have you told your partner what you like sexually?
- Do you desire sex with your partner?
- Do you enjoy sex with your partner?
- Do you feel intimate when you touch?
- Is there a flow of love between you?

These questions recap the essentials of this part of the book. Do you feel happy as you answer? If you have a sensation of discomfort do you need to find the wind in your sails to enter unchartered waters? You may occasionally get wet but you get a life – your own. Attending to your inner Self you learn what lies in your heart. You also learn about your partner and you can each make respectful choices.

I know how difficult it is to update childhood learning, to be able to discuss with respect, to discover your Self and to share this with another. I have accompanied many couples as they talked through the storms of their relationships. I have navigated my own troubled waters. But I have also experienced the personal fulfilment of those who persist in their effort.

As a therapist my own beliefs are frequently challenged. I re-evaluate my thinking in a variety of ways. One of these is to write in a journal. I find it easier sometimes to write a story that represents how I feel.

In the months after I left my marriage I wrote about my own challenges. I bravely sailed into independence. Sometime later I began a new relationship. It was delightful, but I had not found my Self sufficiently and still behaved out of habit. I was still willing to compromise my Self to have a partner. But I did recognise what I was doing. I chose to chart new waters. I gained new awareness, spending time reading, in therapy, soul-searching, having massages and talking with dear friends. Most of all, I walked the beach near my home. In the silence of the beauty I saw and breathed in I found the courage to be my Self.

This story is from my journal. The theme of 'Red Shoes' recurs in legends and fairy tales, but I did not consciously recall these tales as I wrote. This simply welled up from my subconscious.

The Red Shoes

I had always wanted red, peep-toe shoes. Nothing else would do. So I tramped the pavements in bare feet.

Over time my feet became ragged and sore. Occasionally I tried on a pair of shoes but they were discarded as none were right. They were not red, peep-toe shoes. I would take them off carefully and continue to walk the rough pavements. Once again my feet would become sore.

One day when I could walk no further I found a pair of black-lace up shoes. I put them on. They were comfortable and sensible, everyone said so. I walked along in them, relieved that I did not have to feel the impact of the pavement. But I began to look down at my feet and felt twinges of disappointment. I tried dyeing the shoes red. But that wore off. Then I cut a hole in the toes of the shoes but the raw leather rubbed against me. My feet became very sore. Eventually I had to take the shoes off.

Barefoot again I stepped onto a beach. But the sand was hot and burnt the soles of my feet. There before me lay a pair of red, peep-toe shoes. I was excited and rushed to put them on. Now I could walk anywhere. Back on the pavements I skipped along admiring my shoes. But my feet became uncomfortable, the new shoes had caused blisters and made my feet sore. They were too small. I tried to stretch them, but still they hurt. I could not bear to leave them behind, they were very red. But they kept on rubbing my feet.

I tried soaking my feet in cold water. Then I could wear the shoes for a while. But soon my feet would swell back to their original size. My feet would again be sore.

I became fed up with my sore feet.

I took off the red shoes and placed them in a cupboard. I thought about them often. A few weeks later, weary after pacing the streets I opened the cupboard door, took out the red shoes and slipped them on. They looked very beautiful. For a while they felt fine but, of course, the old soreness returned.

I took them off and walked to the beach. I walked until I found cool soft sand. I played in and out of the water enjoying the comfort of my feet.

One day I hope to share the cool sand with another pair of ....comfortable feet.

Part Five

The Shores of the Heart

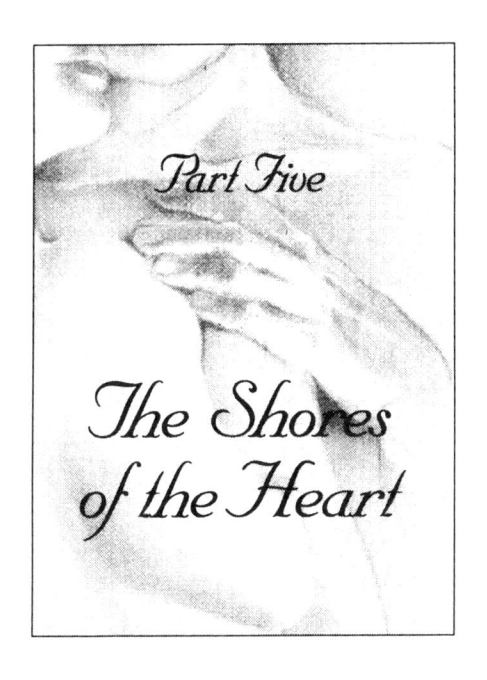

Life is an ocean, love is a boat,
In troubled waters it keeps us afloat.
Our true destination is not marked on any chart.
We're navigating for the shores of the heart.

'The Voyage'
Johnny Duhan

*We have so little faith in the ebb and
flow of life, of love, of relationships.
We leap at the flow of the tide
and resist in terror its ebb.
We insist on permanency,
on duration, on continuity.
When the only continuity possible,
in life as in love, is in growth,
in fluidity — in freedom.*

'Gift from the Sea'[17]
Anne Morrow Lindbergh

Chapter Fifteen

Ebb and flow

The desire for love and sex takes you on a continuing voyage, one that will encounter troubled waters. But you learn to navigate the storms to find your Self charting new waters. You are carried along in the natural flow of a relationship. Eventually though you reach the shores of your heart where you can at last anchor the love boat. You touch down on the shore lapped by the waves of love. A respectful relationship can enrich and nourish you to make ongoing discoveries about your Self in this new land. Your beloved shipmate may also be encountering their inner Self.

At times in harmony, at times in opposition, the connection between you will naturally ebb and flow. When you live openly as your Self you have the strength to appreciate that the other's moods are a reflection of them. They are not about you. Personal integrity provides the solid ground from which you can observe and learn about another. You find the empathy to understand and the independence to know what you like and dislike in the thinking and behaviour of another. You have the freedom to discuss all these aspects of each other with respect. Acceptance of another rather than compromise of your Self becomes possible. You have the clarity of mind to choose what you want in love, in sex, in a partner.

Some aspects of your outer self you like, some you do not. Some you want to change. Some you rejoice in. That is the ebb and flow of your own life. To do this in the presence of a beloved is a most challenging voyage. When two people decide to be together on the shores of their hearts in open honesty, in love and respect they discover new levels of intimacy.

Intimate desires

David Schnarch[18] describes the intimacy of revealing who you are:

Self-validated intimacy sounds like 'I want to be known before I die. It would be nice if you agreed with me, wonderful if you liked me. But most of all I want to know that somebody really knew who and what I am. More than I fear your rejection I fear never reaching across my mortality which separates me from you and others. I will care for my own feelings. Just know me.'

This desire to be known and loved for who you are can be elegantly expressed through sexuality. The communication of sex allows you to display much of what lies within you. In your actions, your heart and mind can be revealed when words may not fully describe how you feel.

When you allow someone to see you inside and out, you may feel vulnerable. But the joy overcomes any previous insecurity that tempted you to hide away your thoughts, feelings and body. When you feel good from the inside you can stand naked and expose your tender strength. You trust your own instincts to do this, having chosen someone whom you like and love.

David Schnarch also writes, 'Love is a concern for the other as well as Self.'

Concern does not now demand the Self sacrifice or unhealthy compromise you have outgrown. It is an acknowledgement of your choice to connect with another for mutual benefit.

Elena and Angelo wanted to know each other more fully. Over the years they had weathered many storms. They were respectful and desirous of each other. But there had been a limit to their expression of this. They were ready to explore the shores of their hearts.

Elena (54) was born in Argentina. Her family migrated to Australia when she was aged 10. She was number five of nine children. Angelo (60) was also Argentinian but migrated to Australia when he was 21. They met at a display of South American folk dancing. They contributed to my thoughts as I wrote some of the earlier parts of this book. But they were stuck on one issue. One I could help them to review. Over the years they respectfully discussed most of their problems, except sex. They had been referred to see me by a Catholic priest. Angelo and Elena had attended his weekend retreat on the joy of sex.

Sitting erect Angelo began:

"*Elena and I have been married for 30 years. We love each other and have a wonderful marriage but sex has never been right. I persuaded Elena to attend the course. I thought as it was run by a priest, that she would listen.*"

Angelo's eyes softened as they lighted on Elena. She squeezed his hand and took a deep breath.

"*I was uncomfortable at first, but what Father Michael said made sense to me. The weekend turned out to be marvellous. All these years I lived with the fear that sex was a sin. Father Michael had a more enlightened view. For the first time I saw that sex could be beautiful. Now I want to enjoy sex but I am still too scared to do so. The biggest problem is it hurts to have sex. It always has.*"

Withdrawing her hand, Elena slipped back into the chair.

"*I never want to hurt Elena. She is so fragile. I just want to love and protect her. I don't press for sex. In fact, we don't do it very often though* sometimes I would really like to. I have always respected Elena. I let things go really. I wouldn't want to upset her. I love her. The sex side has been a bit of a disappointment but nothing else has so I don't complain. She is really reserved about her body. You know she doesn't like me to touch her genitals."

Elena hid her head in her hands and blushed.

"I'm sorry to talk about it, darling. Are you alright?" Angelo asked.

"He's always been tender when we er..." attempted Elena.

"You mean 'make love' darling." Angelo patted her hand.

"Mmn... Yes. I didn't know how to say it."

"It's O.K. don't distress your self. We know what you mean." Angelo stroked her shoulder.

They had compassion for each other. But I could see how Angelo eased Elena's burden – by taking it away from her. He had done so over 30 years of protecting her feelings. Not only did he finish her sentences when she struggled for words, she did not have to face the sex problem for herself.

I asked Elena how she felt about the way Angelo cared for her.

"It makes my life easier and feels safer. Sometimes I'd wish Angelo would let me do more for myself."

I wondered why she had never said so?

"I'm scared I'd do the wrong thing," Elena admitted.

Angelo came to understand that for Elena to grow and become a fully mature woman he needed to stop taking care of her. She needed to take full responsibility for her Self. They recognised the advance they might both make in caring **about** each other rather than taking care **of** each other.

The reasons why each had established this pattern over the years was rooted in learning which dated from childhood. Both needed to update some beliefs.

Angelo had been brought up to care for women as the weaker sex. This made him feel strong. It gave him a secure feeling. Would he be willing to face a woman if he saw her as strong as himself? Or himself as 'vulnerable' as her?

Elena's problem was also tied with her past.

"My Dad was unfair in many ways. He always liked my elder sister better than me. She was pretty and outgoing. I was a mouse. He favoured her and ignored me, except when I did something wrong. Then he'd hit me.

"He was so strong particularly on morals. When I was 13 he shouted at me, in front of my Australian friends for wearing tight shorts. He told me I was a whore and made me go and change. I was stunned. It didn't make sense in Australia. I never knew what to do to be right, with Dad. Things that seemed normal to me were so wrong to Dad. I didn't have any confidence in my self.

"When he found out I'd been kissing boys, he dragged me to confession and the priest lectured me on mortal sin for 45 minutes. I grew up thinking sex was dirty. I never touched my genitals. I never tried tampons. Ugh! I couldn't."

This disgust for her own body had resulted from religious dogma imposed by her father. He had ruled her life. His shadow was still influencing her.

"After the weekend workshop. I gained a new perspective. It reinforced what I had been thinking for a while. Maybe Dad was wrong in this. I want to make my own decision."

Elena was reassessing the ingrained belief that sex was dirty. In her heart she knew it was not, but had not found the courage to face this before. Angelo's acceptance of their limited sex life had not challenged her to grow.

For Angelo, at one level, it had been comfortable for him to accept the status quo. He felt responsible for Elena. He liked to be needed. But he also wanted a closer sexual life with Elena. They were both eager to face one more challenge. Elena was determined to overcome the result of the many years of ingrained fear of sex as sin. To do this she also had to deal with her father's disapproval.

Elena came to see me on her own to talk about her relationship with her father. As he was still alive she decided to deal with an immediate concern.

"*He lives near us. He's 85 and I still do what he tells me. It's ridiculous. I don't give in like this with anyone else. I offered to take him shopping on Thursdays, my day off from work. He insisted I go on Wednesdays. I altered my work roster to please him.*

"*I don't have a lot of spare time. When I arrive he keeps me waiting for an hour. He does it every week. When my sister takes him out he's dressed and ready to go on time. I've had enough of his behaviour.*"

Elena decided to respect herself and discuss this game she and her father played. She had it in her power to change the situation. She returned when she had talked with him.

"*It wasn't easy. I told him if he wasn't ready when I came I'd wait for no more than 10 minutes. I've said that before but always waited longer. After 10 minutes he wasn't ready so I got up to leave. He asked me 'where do you think you're going.' He told me I was too impatient to wait for an old man. He moaned that 'it isn't too much to ask my daughter to take me out once in a while.'*

"*I finally said what I wanted. I was angry but it was like a cold strength. I told him, 'I am willing to take you out but I'm not willing to play this game any more. I'll come back next Wednesday at 2.00 p.m. If you are ready I'll happily take you. If not, I'll leave. Then I left. Ooh! I was shaking inside. What if he complained to my sister about me? But then I thought – 'he does that anyway.'*"

A wave of relief flowed from Elena.

I had my fingers crossed whilst I waited to hear what happened on her next visit with her father. Sometimes it's hard as a therapist to wait until the client gets through their story. Luckily Elena was busting to tell me.

"He was ready on time and do you know he was polite to me." Elena sat tall.

Elena had identified the effect of her overbearing father on her own behaviour. She had wanted to please him to gain his love but did not obtain his respect. She had lived by his standards that made women's sexuality wrong. Now she was being her Self in his presence. She began to do so with Angelo.

Angelo stopped treating her as a child. Elena took responsibility for her Self.

"You know it feels so good to have Elena stand up for herself. If I try to finish her sentence she reminds me not to. It is a relief for me that she has stood up to her father. I used to sympathise with Elena when her Dad was rude but I felt angry inside that she didn't sort him out, nor would she let me say anything. She's becoming quite a woman. I love her even more."

As Elena increased in confidence they felt ready to consider how to improve their sex life. Elena felt unsure about where to start. Elena had not allowed her Self to enjoy the sensuality of her life. Angelo had also closed down awareness of some of his pleasure. He did this to avoid getting turned on 'too easily'.

It was important for them to rediscover the sensual delights of life.

Sensuality

There are five physical senses, hearing, smell, taste, sight and touch. You may also be aware of a sixth sense, that of intuition. With these senses you perceive the surrounding world and your place in it. The sensuality of sex can be delightful. But are you tuned in to receive the information?

To avoid total confusion from too much sensory input you have the ability to pick out the information that you need and ignore the rest. If you are working in an office on a busy road you soon learn to ignore the sound of the traffic.

However, in this modern world you may also be deprived of noticing pleasurable sensory stimulation by your busy-ness. If you are driven by the desire for doing, achieving and accumulating wealth, you can lose contact with the everyday pleasures of the natural world. It is as though you are wearing blinkers and do not sense your surroundings. Focused on future gains you may miss out on the sensual joys of the here and now. Your senses are deadened.

I remember living in a city, working long hours, rushing around performing life. Since altering my perspective I see crimson-breasted honeyeaters in the grevilleas outside my office window. Later I feel the touch of raindrops on my cheek, see the colours of a rainbow and hear the sound of the waves pounding the beach. All in one day.

If you deprive your self of sensual input and instead become a creature of 'doing', life becomes purely practical and dull. I remember asking a Japanese businessman visiting Australia how he spent his Sunday in Japan. It was his only day off work each week.

"At 6.30 a.m. I get up, I go to the bathroom and I brush my teeth. At 6.45 a.m. I switch on the television and watch the news. At 7.00 a.m. I go to the kitchen and have breakfast with my wife. At 7.15 a.m. we wash up the dishes. At 7.30 a.m. I have a shower, get dressed and go for a walk. At 8.00 a.m. I come back from my walk. At 8.30 a.m. I go to the shop and buy the newspapers. I then sit down and read the newspapers."

He proceeded to explain his day in quarter or half-hourly intervals.

I asked if he did the same every Sunday and he answered, 'always.'

Was he performing life, an actor on stage going through the motions? To some extent we all do this in our modern world. Do you find time while walking, not just to go from A to B, but to notice what lies between A and B? To smell, to stop and touch, to sit and feel. Do you turn on music only while doing something else or can you sometimes sit and absorb the sound and allow your Self to drift with the images created.

To enjoy the sensory pleasure of everyday life is part of being alive. Smelling the flowers, gazing on a beautiful scene or painting, listening to music or the sound of the waves, tasting fresh food, stroking a cat – all these and more awaken your body and your inner Self to pleasure.

To be turned on sexually you need to be turned onto life. Then your senses are always at play. When you smell your lover, taste a kiss, savour the sight of your beloved naked, touch skin against skin or feel close, your experience is part of the cycle of awareness. It is more difficult to turn on your senses just to sex when they have been turned off during the rest of the day.

You can awaken your senses with sex but if this is the only time you tap into sensory awareness, you are expecting a great deal from sex. You are presuming that genital touch is powerful enough to first free you from your day-to-day armour and stimulate you sexually. If you allow your senses instead to remain switched on, you soak up simple sensations during the whole day. You thus create a storehouse of good feelings. Feeling good leaves you open to feeling sexy.

Greg and Pauline were busy people but they continued to see me occasionally. Each tended to make an appointment as a new challenge arose. Pauline came to talk about sex.

"I'm so busy with the children and study that I'm still tired. I know Greg would like sex more often. He doesn't pressure me these days but

he does tell me when he would like sex. But I'm beginning to think I'm the one who is missing out! It's just not easy to find time for sex."

I wondered if she found time for her Self.

"I feel guilty taking time out for me when there's so much to do. I'd love to spend some time having a massage or taking time over a meal but I still can't. I know we talked in the sessions about Self sacrifice, I know I still do it. But not half as much as before."

Pauline had certainly made improvement in reducing Self sacrifice. However, being normal, she was finding it takes time to make readjustments in behaviour to find a comfortable balance. I wondered whose voice was saying, 'you can't.' Often this, 'you shouldn't, it's self indulgent' voice is not your own.

"I think I still listen to what Mum and Dad taught me. I guess I don't allow myself much enjoyment. I could try. I would really love to 'smell the roses'. It seems like a dream but we've come so far I want to feel really alive. How do I make that dream come true?"

You have to decide on your own priorities even when you have children. Of course, having a dependent baby reduces your choices. But once children are growing do you contribute to their continuing dependency by taking care **of** them, rather than **about** them? Will you allow your self not to be a 'super Mum or Dad' and respect your own needs as well as those of your children?

To fulfil your dreams in your sexual relationships, you might imagine that a simple (and quick) suggestion for a romantic dinner with candlelight, nice wine and food is all you need to guarantee further sexual activity. But if this is in isolation from sensual awareness to the rest of the day, it is hard for sex to flow on.

It is easy to say, 'I don't have time to stop/smell/look/feel.' Then what do you value? Do you want your life to be consumed by constant doing or will you allow time to open your senses to pleasure?

It is possible to do this in small everyday ways without allocating huge chunks of time. In your office or home your eyes can light on photographs of a beautiful place you visited, fresh flowers can erupt from a vase or a favorite painting can adorn a wall. Your skin can be brushed with silk as you walk and gentle music can soothe you. Your bedroom can be a place of sanctuary away from the children and away from the modern world. When you wake up your day can begin by being stimulated with smells that lighten your mood – your favourite soaps and shampoos in the bathroom, the touch under your feet of a sheepskin rug. Or are you quick to dismiss such 'indulgence' as impossible in your life?

If your whole day is busy full of 'doing' you may benefit by taking some regular breaks. Every hour or so stop for a minute or two. In this time you can focus one of your senses totally on one object you like. You might close your eyes and just use your ears to listen to the birds singing outside, or close your ears and use your eyes to look at a picture. These sensory breaks help to relieve stress levels and is a reminder of life beyond the 'doing' of the office, children, cooking or shopping.

If your day has been very full with 'doing', when you first come home, take some time to go for a walk or sit in the garden or sit in a chair and play some gentle music. At first this may require effort. Eventually, you wonder how you could ever have been so isolated from enjoying sensations.

Pauline found she enjoyed the return of sensual awareness to her life. She and Greg wanted some assistance in expanding everyday sensuality through to sexuality.

"We've both been busy working, raising children. With sex being a problem it was easier to focus on other parts of life. I erected a barrier between loving and sex, now I want to overcome that," Pauline began.

"I'm knocked out that Pauline is raising the issue of sex rather than me. But I'm interested too. I'd also like sex to be more relaxed. I suppose we have tried to squeeze sex in between everything else. I think being happy is a priority. I'm beginning to feel there is much more we can do in this direction for ourselves." Greg nodded thoughtfully.

To stimulate their thinking to allow sensuality to flow onto sexuality I started a short 'sensual/sexy' list with a few basic ideas. I suggested they add their own ideas. You may find this useful also. Consider each of your senses and see what appeals to you. The only limits are your imagination. If you do this individually at first, it can be fun to share later.

This is the combination of their separate lists:

Sensual/sexy list

Visual
- moonlight
- sunrise
- paintings
- the colour of the bedroom
- wearing sexy underwear
- seeing her in sexy underwear
- him naked, particularly his bum
- my breasts
- nude pictures

....
....
....

Smell
- fresh bread
- perfumed flowers
- wearing my favourite scent

- ❧ his aftershave
- ❧ freshly washed sheets
- ❧ wood shavings
- ❧ her vagina

Taste
- ❧ sweet strawberries
- ❧ wine
- ❧ ice cream coated with chocolate
- ❧ skin saltiness
- ❧ her vagina
- ❧ inside her mouth
- ❧ tip of his penis

Touch
- ❧ fur
- ❧ vibrator
- ❧ feathers
- ❧ cuddling
- ❧ kissing
- ❧ stroking
- ❧ having my hair brushed
- ❧ being touched on the breasts
- ❧ a gentle touch in passing.
- ❧ giving a massage
- ❧ my clitoris

- my penis
- inside her vagina
- my G spot
- inner thighs
- all over
- around my anus

....

....

Intuitive
- I feel close to him
- intimacy
- I just want to
- why not?
- sharing a tender moment
- telling you what I like
- having the courage to show you my body
- letting you know what I'm thinking

....

....

It can be a surprise to read what your partner likes. The things you both like are easy. How do you feel about what your partner likes but you have not shared before? There is no compulsion to do what your partner wants. You know what you like to do and can now open your mind to what you have not thought of before. Adding the intuitive sense to sensuality opens another dimension of your Self in sexuality. If you find at times you are both aroused by sensuality, sex can flow on. This combination of talking, touching and loving forms the sexual intimacy of a couple grown beyond their previous limits:

*Our bodies open
you with ease
me with reserve
the challenge of shared intimacy.
You enter my body
not in conquest
but from desire
to know me.
I reveal my Self.
You come inside me.*

*Our minds open
you with reserve
me with ease
the challenge of shared intimacy.
I enter your mind
not in conquest
but from desire
to know you.
You reveal your Self.
I come inside you.*

*This difference between us
an opportunity.
I learn through you
what is incomplete in me.
You learn through me
what is incomplete in you.
Two aspects of intimacy
understood by contrast.
Embracing both
each becomes whole.*

'Intimate lovers'

D.S.

There is no goal involved in sharing your sensuality with your partner. The sharing is an intimation of love that sometimes contains the surprise of your partner becoming turned on.

You can equally savour the times when you or your partner are not aroused to sex but prefer a quieter togetherness or simply move away to be alone at that time. That is the ebb and flow of a comfortable sexual relationship.

Pauline and Greg needed to overcome the barrier between sensuality and sexuality to enjoy this easier flow. They found making the sexy/sensual list helped them do so.

"It was fun. I laughed when he told me he feels sexy if I bake bread. I had visions of having sex on the kitchen table covered in flour." Pauline grinned at the recollection.

" I got turned on just making the list," laughed Greg.

"It feels different to feel turned on in myself and then share this with Greg. It used to be the other way round. I'd try to feel sexy to please him and that never felt completely right," Pauline added.

The tension had disappeared from talking about sex for Greg and Pauline. They were enjoying their relationship. Each had expanded their involvement in intimacy valuing both the physical and talking aspects.

Elena and Angelo had also been taking significant strides since Elena had released herself from the sexual oppressiveness of her childhood. Not only had she updated her beliefs on sexuality but she had become Self assured since respecting her Self with her father.

"I don't think we have a sexual problem now. We have a passion that we want to fulfil," Angelo ventured.

Elena needed some help at first with suggestions for relaxation. She enjoyed using a tape I made for her with pleasant imagery of unwinding in her favourite place. She found she not only relaxed her body but also allowed her mind to play. Sometimes the images were spontaneously sexy and she enjoyed this. She and Angelo had made their own sensual/sexy list, which helped them to talk more freely about their desires. They had also enjoyed reawakening their senses in the everyday.

Elena and Angelo were delighted to have taken the sharing of sexuality beyond its previous limits.

"Elena is becoming braver. She even called me up this week at work and said she 'wanted' me. But she knew I was busy – the minx. I fixed her though. I got in the car and drove home, there and then. I thought, 'After I run my own business, I can please myself.' I wasn't sure how she'd take it but she was pleased. We made love all afternoon."

Elena had a naughty smile. *"I enjoyed it too. There was no pain. I think the cream you recommended really helped."*

The hormone cream I had prescribed would certainly have relieved the discomfort caused by thinning skin of her vagina associated with menopause. But I thought the magic had come from inside Elena as she emerged from the shadow of her father and Angelo and became her own woman.

Elena and Angelo continued to open up their sexual pleasure with each other. Both became comfortable with touching the other intimately. Each felt excited if this led them to intercourse and relaxed when it did not. Gradually, Angelo challenged Elena with sexual suggestions expanding what they did and where.

Elena was using her own imagination.

"We were on holiday in the countryside. I was feeling sexy when we were out walking. I told Angelo and he was excited too. We found a private place in the tall grass beside a river. I felt completely relaxed and uninhibited. It was so sexy."

Angelo and Elena had a robust relationship. They were both open to change and delighted in the other gaining in stature. Growth was not only occurring in their sexual life.

Many months later Elena returned to see me.

"I had felt angry after that weekend workshop. I felt stupid and immature for still believing what my Dad and the Church had told me when I was young. I hated my Dad for a while. But I still loved him.

"He became frail recently after a bout of the 'flu and I nursed him. I asked him about his own early years and realised he had had a hard life himself. I forgave him. He had a heart attack a week ago. I rushed to the hospital. No one else from the family had arrived. He looked terrible but he could speak. 'I'm glad you're here Elena,' he said. I took his hand and replied 'I love you Dad.'

"He closed his eyes and slipped into unconsciousness. He died an hour later. I was still holding his hand."

Elena had in those last few months completed her unfinished business from childhood. She had been lucky enough to have reached out to her father and respected her Self. She had become whole.

"Angelo and I are closer than ever and sex is so special now. We are completely open with each other. I even fantasised about sex with Angelo the other day." She still blushed. *"I think Father Michael was right – sexuality is a gift of love from God."*

The world of fantasy...
The abundant, hilarious, naughty,
healing, evocative lives we can lead in our heads.

'Burning Urges'[19]
Ruth Ostrow

Chapter Sixteen

Skinny dipping

The voyage has its challenges and through troubled waters you may have lost contact with the fun you had when you first embarked. On the shores of your heart, fun returns to loving. You feel like throwing your clothes off and skinny-dipping in the warm blue water, making love with abandon, then basking in the sun. Love and sex can be exciting!

Erotica or pornography?

Our culture, however, holds deeply rooted fears about freedom, particularly if it is sexual. It is feared that you could not possibly handle all that choice. There is a suspicion that unbridled freedom in sex would lead to orgies at the very least. But does an orgy sound like freedom or a desperate search? Freedom of choice requires mature thinking whereas prohibition is more likely to stimulate an unthinking child-like drive to taste forbidden fruit.

Most people I counsel value love and sex with a known chosen partner. It is when their relationship is in troubled waters they are more likely to have a sexual affair, not as a result of a natural easy freedom but often as an escape from unresolved problems.

It is sad that our culture has often failed to differentiate between erotica and pornography. What is erotic for one, may initiate a negative feeling in another. This quote reveals a common way to distinguish the two by applying a very personal standard and assuming that to be an absolute truth.

> *I cannot define what material is obscene. But I know what it is when I see it.*
>
> Potter Stewart, Supreme Court Judge US, 1964

We separate erotica from pornography but not every one has the same interpretation.

> *Attempts to sort out good erotica from bad pornography inevitably come down to what turns me on is – what turns you on (if different) is pornographic.*
>
> Ellen Willis, staff writer, Village Voice

I use two definitions. I realise these are open to interpretation by an individual or culture.

Erotica: sexually stimulating and respectful of the integrity of others.

Pornography: sexually stimulating in association with the misuse of power. It is demeaning to the object of arousal.

It is respect that clearly separates erotica from the disrespect inherent in pornography. The use of a child, who can never be consenting, in a sexual relationship with an adult is pornographic. The depiction of a person in some way entrapped, denigrated, debased by another, for me, is pornographic. The consent of an adult, in loving respect of them Self with another, in any aspect of their sexuality, is erotic. Yet we have developed a cultural standard that erotic is dirty. How can you respectfully explore your sexual potential? As you seek to please your Self and honour your partner you still can open to new ideas.

Pushing beyond your limitations can enhance sexual joy. There are many experiences which stimulate you into a fuller awareness of your sexual being.

Genital touch is an obviously erotic source of stimulation. But much erotic awareness uses other senses such as reading books with a sexual content, dancing to music that stirs the mind and the body. Flamenco particularly comes to mind in this respect. Other experiences like skinny dipping, letting your eyes linger on luscious photographs – any of these and many more can be erotic. New positions, awareness of all of the body, stimulating extras such as silk, feather and vibrators can be explored when you feel equal to express not only your desires but also your dislikes. Sharing the content of your heart and mind in fun, in fantasy, in love, in honesty can also be erotic. You will notice that these appear in the 'sensual/sexy list' (page 247) as there need be no separation into erotic, sexy or sensual categories. One simply flows into another dependent on mutual consent.

For centuries books, such as the *Kama Sutra*, have existed full of suggestions for erotic exploration. With a solid sense of Self you do not feel naughty when you pick up an erotic book in the shop. You even have the confidence to ask the assistant, looking him/her straight in the eyes, directions to the erotic book section. As you browse you can choose for your Self what does or does not appeal to you.

An erotic experience is one that stimulates and enhances your sexual turn-on or arousal. The obvious is well catered for by the enormous number of erotice magazines and videos offering visual stimulation. Unfortunately, few respect the equality of man and woman in sexuality. Much of the focus is on physical senses. Awareness of inner Self or feelings of the heart are often ignored. Body, mind and spirit can be part of sexual pleasure. All can be stimulated and enlivened as you become more aware, not only of your Self but also of your partner. This broader view is beginning to be presented in some books and videos.[20]

The setting can also contribute to the erotic content of sex. An edge of excitement that many young people experience early on their voyage of sexual exploration can so easily be lost by 'settling down' to the routine of life aboard the love boat. It can be fun to become adventurous again.

Sex on deck, in the water, sex in rooms other than your cabin can all be part of spontaneous desire and add to sexual sharing. Lightheartedness can be very sexy.

What is erotic for you? What repulses you about sexuality? How do you share these desires and fears with your beloved? The more you know your inner Self the clearer your answers become.

You may recognise that your partner has different limits to you. You discover what these are when you are willing to expose your desires to each other. It is not that you should give in to every request of your partner but that you be willing to listen, attempt to understand and consider the possibility of expanding. To do this you need to reflect on why you have a taboo in the first place. Has your view been implanted by someone else or is it truly your own? It is for you to decide what you want to do with your body and how you wish to physically express your desire with your partner.

What turns you on? With Self esteem you choose for your Self what you wish to do sexually. There are no assumptions that your partner should comply as a proof of love. You become willing to say what your interests and desires are and respect your differences. This may involve excitement and disappointment, new challenges and new joys.

Fantasy

One of the popular suggestions to spice up your sex life is to try to fantasise. It has become the latest thing you 'should' do to be sexually modern. The more unusual and outrageous the better. Or is it?

Distraction

Fantasy can be a distraction. We know women in the Victorian era were encouraged to indulge in the fantasy of 'lie back and think of England' to be able to tolerate sex. This is often the role fantasy fulfils when you are in troubled waters.

If you are not enjoying sex with your partner you may use fantasy to become aroused. If you can only become turned on when your mind is totally absorbed on being admired and made love to by a film star, you have found a way to make sex tolerable with your partner. But the fantasy distances you from your partner. Distractive fantasy is like bailing out water from your sinking boat with a small bucket. Your sexual relationship will stay afloat a bit longer but still sink if you do not fix the cause of the leak.

Sexual pleasure is not just about genital touch but about the opening of your Self to include your imagination with your body. Fantasy can expand you or be no more than a band-aid for a troubled relationship. Fantasy can be just one more quick fix to avoid dealing with underlying problems of intimacy.

Sam Keen[21] was asked to write an article on the first legal public sex club, which opened in New York City in 1979 called Plato's Retreat. He reported that the club was a sanctuary where people might explore sensation divorced from feeling. He described the couples playing out their fantasies as 'disembodied genitals in search of romance.' I was struck by the sadness of this observation of sexual loneliness. In a different state of mind, sexual fantasy can be an intimate sharing.

Knowledge

The content of fantasy is formed in your mind and can illuminate your hopes and fears. It may be framed around real events or people or have the bizarre nature of dreams.

Bringing these thoughts to the surface of your mind does have value. You can decide what the meaning is for you. You can learn about your Self. If you compose images of dominance over another or inflicting/receiving pain, your mind is focused back in the dark depths of win/lose. Such fantasy may well come from a part of your psyche that you may consider could benefit from a review and update.

If you choose to share the content of your fantasy with your partner you are revealing a part of your Self. Your partner learns more about you. Sharing a fantasy can allow you to know and be known.

Fun

Of course, there are the more light-hearted, fun-filled fantasies that lift your spirit. Playing is not just for children.

Acting out your fantasy involving another is a decision for two people. If you maintain an open mind you can decide what you feel is respectful of your Self.

When you have a mature love there can be true sexual fireworks. When you and your beloved have honest open communication, you say whatever you think and feel – including sexually. Limits and sexual boundaries become more fluid than in Provisional Love. It feels OK to make a suggestion and to hear either a negative or positive response from your partner. In mature love you can share the erotic images that come into your mind in the form of sexual fantasies. Fantasy then is not a distraction. Greg and Pauline came back after a few months to update me on how they were going. They had moved a long way since their early sessions.

They were delighted to share a recent discussion they had had on fantasy.

"Greg told me his fantasy and wanted to act it out. I was not sure how I felt. I enjoy sex now. I'm more relaxed and am taking care of my self. So is Greg. But he had an idea that made me feel nervous."

I asked if what Greg suggested had felt wrong to her.

"No. But I felt a tightness in my stomach. My first reaction was to say 'No'. But I gave myself a few minutes to think. I decided I needed to talk this through with Greg. How we talked was good."

I asked them to recreate their conversation. This had been a challenge and I was interested as to how they had handled it.

Greg had started by saying what he wanted to do.

"I would like to tie you to the bed and have sex with you," Greg stated clearly.

" I'd like to understand why." Pauline invited.

Pauline had opened her mind to listen to Greg rather than prejudging him.

"I'd feel powerful like a caveman. Like Tarzan beating my chest."

Greg expanded his chest and looked most imposing.

Greg was being honest about a primitive, strongly masculine urge inside himself. But was this his only reason?

"I can understand, but I feel scared about being tied. Being physically tied down would limit my ability to stop at any time. You'd be in control." Pauline responded in a steady voice.

Pauline accepted Greg's view but also expressed her own.

" I must admit I hadn't really thought about why I wanted to. But that could be part of my reason. But it does turn me on to think about it," Greg grinned.

"How would you feel if I tied you up and had twice your physical strength like you have compared to me?" Pauline offered.

She invited Greg to put himself in her position.

"*Shit scared!*"

They both started laughing. But they continued to talk.

"*I'd like to give that primitive bit a go. If you want to be Tarzan I'll be Jane. But I don't want to be tied up.*"

They had made a light hearted adjustment that suited them both and presented an opportunity for further knowing of each other.

I asked Pauline how she felt about their discussion.

"*When Greg first suggested it, I thought I don't want to know. But then I knew he was being open with me. Before I made a decision I realised I did want to know more.*"

I asked Greg how he felt about Pauline saying 'No' to being tied up.

"*Some disappointment at first because I wanted to. But when she asked me to put myself in her position my response of being scared came from my guts. Then I didn't want to tie her up. I didn't feel what we said was wrong. Talking made us both think. I remembered all the problems that wanting control had caused. I've come to realise that understanding and being understood is more important.*"

This response came from mature love with respect. I wondered how their fantasy game worked out.

"*I started out as Tarzan. It was fun. We both enjoyed playing around. She was seeing this basic erotic part of me. Then I looked in her eyes and saw she was fearless. Suddenly I knew I didn't want to dominate her. I wanted to touch her, softly. And I did.*" They exchanged a knowing smile.

If you want to play out a fantasy with your partner you each have an equal say in what happens. But what you say must be honest. You are on the very edge of facing your own doubts and fears. Do you want to know all of your partner? Fantasy can be a way of sharing the excitement of your own imagination. When approval seeking is no longer part of a relationship then you can say what comes into your mind. Your partner may find it exciting as well or they may not. Sharing a fantasy can be part of a very deep level of intimacy. It is not essential, it is a matter of choice.

When you have open, honest communication, erotic connection can take whatever form you want. At this stage respect for your Self and each other define the limits. These limits, of course, may change as you continue to expand.

~

*When lovers meet with respect for the mystery
of their separateness, they may, in coming together,
suddenly experience lovemaking as a sacramental dance,
an outward and visible sign of the invisible grace,
that unites the single self to the communion of Being.
Only then does sexuality become a path
to wisdom and compassion.*

'Hymns to an Unknown God'
Sam Keen

Chapter Seventeen

Dawn on the horizon

Two people stroll along the shore in the coolness of dawn. You meet and stop to watch the wakening of the day. The sun rises up your legs, caresses your thighs, awakens your genitals, warms your heart and lights up your mind. You feel touched by love and the presence of one who stands beside you.

The love boat is anchored in the bay. Today you may sail to explore some new land, bask in the sun on the shore or face an unexpected storm. Who knows what each day will bring?

But in the midst of the unknown there is the known joy of thriving as your Self and savouring the company of a beloved. You no longer need the relationship but do desire to spend time with a partner for your enjoyment.

You are together from freedom of choice having learned much about your Self and the other on your voyage. A new ease infuses the relationship. You have discovered on the shores of the heart how to live side by side.

A complete sharing between two people is an impossibility and whenever it seems, nevertheless, to exist, it is a narrowing, a mutual agreement which robs either one member or both of his fullest freedom and development.

But once the realisation is accepted that, even between the closest human beings, infinite distances continue to exist, a wonderful living side by side can grow up, if they succeed in loving the distance between them which makes it possible for each to see the other whole against a wide sky.

Rainer Maria Rilke

By this time you have developed a sensitivity in communication with your companion. Your love contains compassion for your partner. In my years of counselling and medicine I have been privileged to meet people who navigated their troubled waters to develop a deep understanding in which being together was no longer based on rules, regulations or contracts, but on desire. As a result their sexuality was an integral part of their open and relaxed connection.

Frank and Lil were two such people. They had been married for 56 years. They had met in an air raid shelter in London in 1942. Their doctor had suggested this sprightly couple come to see me to discuss a physical limitation in sex. Frank had a coronary bypass two years previously. His erections had not been good for about three years.

I listened to the story of their lives together.

"We've had our ups and downs, but we've always loved each other. It has been wonderful to share our lives together. Mind you he can be a miserable old sod sometimes, but then so can I. Nothing serious though. We always managed to sort things out. We just have a rhythm between us that feels good," Lil explained in her sunny cockney accent.

Frank continued, "We worked together, bringing up the kids, keeping food on the table. It was a struggle sometimes. But Lil was always a brick, she mucked in with everything. We both did. Sure we had our disagreements. *She was always so damned honest about her opinions. Sometimes it led to an argument when we disagreed. But we listened to each other. We always respected each other. I've done what I wanted in my life, so has Lil. Because some of that was the same we did some together.*

"We've always enjoyed a cuddle too. That's why we came to see you Doc. You may think it's silly at our age but we've had a good sex life. I'm having some trouble in that department. I read about these injections that men can jab into their 'equipment' and wondered if it would work for me. I thought the erection pills sounded good but they aren't recommended with my heart tablets."

"Now we're retired we enjoy our time together," said Lil. "We're just on a pension but we manage. We can't have intercourse at the moment because he doesn't get hard like. We still play around and that's fun but if it was possible to fix him up I'd like that." Lil had a definite twinkle in her eye.

I explained that if the arteries to his penis were badly blocked the injection may not work. They wanted to give it a try. I injected the first dose to demonstrate how to use it correctly. It worked just fine.

"There's life in the old dog yet." Frank beamed from ear to ear.

Lil decided that she would be better at giving the injection than Frank, at home.

"His eyesight is hopeless. I put in his eyedrops for him so I can do this too."

"I may be half blind but I still have my dignity Lil. I thank you for putting in the drops but I'll do the injection. Anyway, if I gave it to you I'd end up like a pin cushion. You know she's still pretty keen." He winked with pride.

The state of grace exuded by these two mature human beings, living together in respect and joy, filled my office and touched my heart for a long time. They obviously found great delight in sharing their voyage.

You do not have to be married for 56 years to know mature love. At any age you can navigate through the limitations and confusions of 'provisional love' and 'dependent love' to release your true Self. This personal freedom overcomes any obstacles to express your Self in words, action, love and sex. Therefore, your sexuality becomes an affirmation of your unique Self, to share your experience with your beloved is an intimate disclosure.

Body/spirit/mind-blowing orgasm

Sex infused with respect is different to sex originating from win/lose conflict. The former has an emphasis on satisfaction of your whole being, the latter only on performance.

Popular magazines, books and sex programmes promote sexual goals. Multiple orgasms, mutual orgasm, G-spot sensations and lasting longer have become the Holy Grail of sex.

There is an illusion these prizes offer a guarantee of sexual happiness. But if you have to struggle to achieve these goals, sex becomes a performance accompanied by a niggling feeling that something is missing, even during orgasm. Both men and women describe the sexual performance that leads to an orgasm, which leaves them feeling 'fine'.

There are differences between the orgasmic response achieved by focusing on a goal and one that spontaneously erupts when you allow the pleasure of sex to ooze through you. The latter is a deeply personal experience that is not dependent, nor totally independent of your lover, but a delightful sharing. This is a different experience – the body/spirit/mind-blowing orgasm. The French call this orgasm 'le petit mort' (the little death) in recognition of the overwhelming nature of this experience.

Many of the words you use to describe a sexual climax are words also used in a spiritual context, 'It was divine', 'heavenly', 'Oh my God!' Orgasm and the following peace can be a time when you fully open to your Self. This comes from the ease of being able to be your Self with your beloved – in all situations. This frees you to the sheer joy of orgasm as a total absorption in the ecstasy of the moment. It leaves an afterglow not to be forgotten.

> We float back to earth
> transfigured by divine light,
> enchantment sustained.
>
> We desire nothing
> but to savour the moment,
> infinite instant.
>
> The stillness lingers
> long after the passion ebbs,
> peace floods our bodies.
>
> We open our selves
> revealing new dimensions,
> sharing beyond words.
>
> Our soul connection
> deepens with each encounter,
> wholeness made richer.

'Afterglow'
Andy Hede

Divine sex

Orgasm can be a delight that transports you from being a totally separate individual to a sense of being part of something greater. A feeling of being connected by love. You expand your sense of your Self in isolation to a view of spiritual wholeness. It is as though the sexual experience sets you resonating.

The sharing of sexual desire has the potential to be fulfilling, satisfying and transcending.

Eastern Tantric practices have acknowledged this spiritual element of sexuality for centuries. But practicing breathing techniques, chanting or special techniques will not, of themselves, impart any special sexual magic. Underlying Tantra and other spiritual practices is participation in the challenging process of attaining Self knowledge and respect of others.

Across the planet there are many different concepts of divinity. Many people have a sense that there is more to human life than merely an animal existence. The feelings of love and compassion seem unique to humanity. You feel it when a survivor is dragged from the ruins of their home destroyed in an earthquake, when your child is born, when you see a glorious sunrise or when you share in sexual communion.

In recent centuries we have been reliant on the neat science of logic to explain ourselves. But even pure scientists confront the inexplicable in our existence.

Everyone who is seriously involved in the pursuit of science becomes convinced that the spirit is manifest in the laws of the universe.
Albert Einstein

It is not necessary to embrace New Age philosophies to be aware of your inner Self. Through the ages our culture has told many tales through the *Bible* and mythology of the importance of Self. A frequent theme of such tales concerns a person tempted by the devil to sell their soul. The bargain is to give up their soul (Self, Spirit) to receive riches which it is promised will make them happy, a fortune, the love of a beautiful woman, a kingdom, whatever their heart desires. The tragedy is that having sold their soul (to the devil) they are not happy.

These tales could well represent the Self sacrifice that you might have made in your own life. A sexual relationship may tempt you to lose your Self. But later on you will not feel fulfilled if you have sold your soul for happiness. Happily, the emerging discomfort of troubled waters later challenges you to grow until you become your whole Self and experience fulfilment.

To be directed by your own inner wisdom after many years of being educated to look outside for happiness is a considerable task. You will find help from books, therapy, workshops and friends but the voyage is your own. Peace and quiet in natural surroundings are often beneficial in navigating this shift in focus. Meditation, walking, swimming, music, stroking your cat – whatever is your way to find relief from the busy chatter of everyday.

After walking on my own in my favourite quiet place recently I made an entry in my journal. I had watched the opsreys soar and then swoop to catch their supper from the ocean. The last rays of sunlight for the day painted a glow across the sky and I felt that life had meaning. These words came from my inner Self.

You must find your Self alone
To know that you are not.

D.S.

In this state of mind, it is a delight to also share this contentment and joy. It can be the core of passion and compassion. As you allow this to flow on to sexuality you can experience an enriching warmth in sexual communion.

Whereas the earlier stages of a relationship can be worked on, to nurture and improve the relationship, communion is a spontaneous reaction. Something that occurs between two people as they stand in their separate joy and recognise they want to share their sensual Selves.

Unconditional touch

This delight of your whole Self is not only experienced during sexual intercourse, there is much more to communion. Sex is no longer an isolated event. Instead it is integrated in the perpetual wave motion of sensuality. Sexual intercourse and orgasm form the crest of the waves that continuously ebb and flow along the shores of your heart.

The gentle waves of love that flow through you can be communicated in unconditional touch. This touch intimates your own pleasure in being close to the one you love. There is no assumption that the touch should stimulate any response. It is sufficient in itself in that moment. Unconditional touch contains no expectation that sex will follow. It is the touch of your body which contains your heart and soul.

When it does spontaneously crest in sexual intercourse it adds another dimension to intimate experience and is yours to treasure in your heart. Words can be inadequate to describe this feeling but when Jackie (page 64) spoke of her love and sex with Paul, she was able to provide them.

"When I wake up in the morning, Paul is still asleep. I lean over and smell his hair. It's liked crushed thyme and lemons. I gently stroke his head. He never stirs. I am filled with tenderness. The day starts with the touch of my love.

"Sex is a continuation of my love. I touch Paul in ways that gives me

a tingle. If he happens to become aroused I may do too. The feeling just flows back and forth between us. Touching each other like that builds naturally. That's how I climax. My orgasm is a celebration of me, my love for Paul and it reaches the depth of my soul. I feel the touch of the divine during sex."

Perhaps after all the trials and tribulations of daily life, graceful sex is a loving gift. One that transports you onto a plain of ecstasy. This is a personal experience that cannot be attained by study alone, you have to be willing to risk living it – just as the peace of meditation comes when you let go of practice and find a deep connection beyond your Self.

I hope that in reading this book you rediscover your deepest resources and realise your dreams. In finding your Self you may also have the pleasure of being known by your Beloved. I hope that through your sexual relationship you too come to celebrate the fulfilment of happiness on your Voyage of Love and Sex.

References

1   *The Naked Ape Trilogy*, Desmond Morris, Johnathan Cape 1994.
2   *Brain Sex* (video), Anne Moir. Premedia Prod. 1992.
3   *Sexuality in Adolescence*, Dr S. Moore, Prof D. Rosenthal. Govt. Pub. 1993.
4   *Show Me Yours*, Ronald & Juliette Goldman. Penguin, 1988.
5, 8   *The Feeling of Healing*, Women's Project Group, P.O. Box 384. Cotton Tree, Qld. 4558.
      Sexual Abuse Services, Crisis/Emergency listing and Personal/Family listing. See White Pages in each state.

6   *Menopause*, Dr Sandra Cabot. WHAS, 1991.
7   *Proceedings of the 13th World Congress of Sexology.* WAS 1997.
9   *Appetites*, Geneen Roth. Penguin, 1996.
10   Suggested Books:
      Good Loving Great Sex, Dr Rosie King. Random House, 1997.
      Women's Experience of Sex, Sheila Kitzinger. Penguin,

References

1985.
11 *Australian Society Sex Educators Researchers Therapists* (ASSERT). See Yellow Pages - 'Counselling'.
12, 13 *The Power of Unconditional Love*, Ken Keyes. Love Line Books, 1990.
14 *The Law of Love*, Laura Esquivel, Random House, 1995.
15 *Emotional Blackmail*, Dr Susan Forward. Bantam Press. 1997.
16 *Mediation Services*, Relationships Australia, and Lifeline.
17 *Gift From the Sea*, Anne Morrow Lindbergh. Vintage, 1991 (orig. 1955).
18 *Constructing the Sexual Crucible*, David Schnarch. Norton, 1991.
19 *Burning Urges*, Ruth Ostrow. Pan Macmillan, 1997.
20 Suggested Videos :
    Sacred Sex I & II. Triple Image Film P/L. Home Cinema Group.
    Suggested Books:
    The Art of Tantric Sex, Nitya La Croix. Penguin 1997.
21 *Hymns to an Unknown God*, Sam Keen. Bantam Books, 1991.

THE VOYAGE OF LOVE & SEX

To order *The Voyage of Love & Sex* mail this coupon to:
Summer Books and Seminars
P.O. Box 224, Moffat Beach, Qld. 4551, Australia

Please send me .... copies of *The Voyage of Love and Sex*
@ AUS $22.95 (plus postage and handling $5.00)

Please charge my credit card (tick correct card)
❏ Bankcard ❏ Mastercard ❏ Visa Card

Expiry date............/...............

Your CREDIT CARD No.
❏❏❏❏ ❏❏❏❏ ❏❏❏❏ ❏❏❏❏

Your Signature..
Your Name...
Your Address...
Postcode...
Telephone...............................Fax...
Email..

Or Order by: Email: summer@a1.com.au
Fax: (07) 5445 3012
Ph: (07) 5437 0357

Please ensure you supply all information for payment and dispatch before mailing.

You may also contact Summer Books and Seminars for details on workshops in your area.